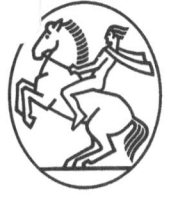

D. Stula

Cranioplasty

Indications, Techniques, and Results

Springer-Verlag Wien New York

Dragoslav Stula, M. D.
Associate Professor, Neurosurgical Clinic, Department of Surgery
University of Basel, Switzerland

With 73 Figures

Library of Congress Cataloging in Publication Data. Stula, D. (Dragoslav), 1939– . Cranioplasty: indications, techniques, and
results. 1. Skull – Surgery. 2. Surgery, Plastic. I. Title. [DNLM: 1. Skull – abnormalities. 2. Skull – surgery. 3. Surgery, Plastic.
WE 705 S934c]. RD529.S85. 1984. 617′.514. 84-10694

ISBN-13:978-3-7091-8764-7   e-ISBN-13:978-3-7091-8762-3
DOI: 10.1007/978-3-7091-8762-3

Foreword

This monograph presents a comprehensive review of the clinical experience in surgical repair of cranial defects which the author has gained during a period of over ten years. Particular problems of patients undergoing cranioplasty, such as neurological impairments, EEG changes, variations of intracranial pressure, and sinking skin flap syndrome are described and discussed.

The author presents convincing evidence of the importance of cranioplasty in improving the quality of life of patients with large and disfiguring cranial defects. Unfortunately, cranioplasty still ameliorates only to a minimal extent the general condition in patients suffering of major cerebral lesions.

I am convinced that this volume will serve the purpose it was designed for: that it will be a most helpful introduction into the problems related to reconstructive surgery.

Basel, August 1984   Otmar Gratzl

Contents

Introduction

Until recently, the influence of cranial defects upon the underlying intracranial structures has not been sufficiently appreciated. The cranial defect was looked upon as a more or less cosmetic problem. Some authors today still adher to the opinion that a cranial bone plastic is performed purely for cosmetic purposes [79, 142, 169]; if, however, other aspects are also relevant, requires a definite answer. Also, a matter of discussion is, which material is the most compatible with the surrounding tissue and last but not least the most practicable. Some authors prefer acrylates [71, 100, 102, 114, 141, 149, 169]. Others [102, 169] still cover cranial defects with metal plates, while a third group uses mainly bony material [4].

There is no consensus about the indication for the cranial closure and the appropriate time to do it. The best time to perform cranioplasty after infections has also not been precisely set. There are few investigations and, therefore, little is known about intracranial changes due to the immediate effect of atmospheric pressure on patients with, in particular, large cranial defects. In the last few years only, thanks to the discovery of cerebral computer tomography, it has become possible to recognize neurological symptoms, psychic changes, headaches and dizziness, as being a consequence of cranial defects [162]. A detailed and continuous analysis of these changes in a large number of patients is not known until today. These problems, however, deserve attention since cranial injuries have drastically increased with the ever increasing number of traffic and industrial accidents. Head injuries represent 70% of all fatal road accidents [30, 104].

Cerebral diagnostics has been remarkably improved by the development of computer tomography [37]. Several pathological intracranial changes (for example: small brain tumours, intracerebral bleeding, and some parasitic brain illnesses) which escaped earlier neuroradiological methods can now be quickly diagnosed with certainty. Due to these reasons the number of craniotomies, together with bone flap decompression, has increased. As a result the plastic covering of skull defects is being more and more performed, and the actual problems in this field deserve a quick solution. However, in the last few years, after the introduction of cerebral oedema treatment with corticosteroids and barbiturate therapy, controlled by cerebral pressure readings, the number of decompression craniotomies has significantly decreased.

Reconstructive cranial bone surgery has recently gained more topical interest in view of the fact that most of the operated brain injuries occur in young people, who need to be quickly integrated into society and professional life again.

The purpose of this review is to determinate the indications, the time to operate, the appropriate operating technique and the best suitable material for the cranioplasty. In addition, we analyzed the effect of cranioplasty on the neurological status and studied the electrical irritability of the brain and the cerebral circulation before and after the closure of the skull defects. Finally, in an attempt to understand the pathophysiological changes in this situation, we undertook continuous intracranial pressure readings before and after the cranioplasty.

A. History of Cranioplasty

Trepanation is probably one of the oldest surgical interventions. It was already performed in the Stone Age [57, 109, 119]. First evidence of this came from a French doctor, Prunières, who found several prehistorical trepanated skulls in the Department Lozère in the south of France in the year 1873 [109, 119, 182]. Today, numerous similar observations have been registrated throughout the whole world.

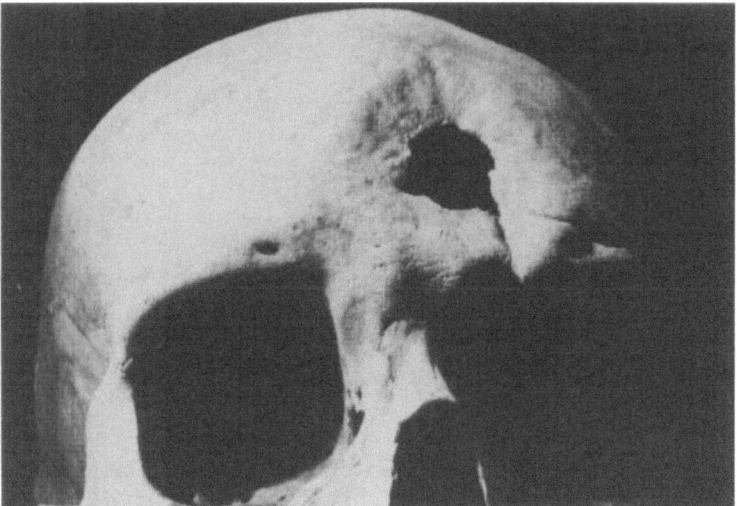

Fig. 1. Trepanation of an Inka skull. Bone regeneration on the edge of the defect indicates that the patient survived the operation

The graveyards of Paracas and Parachamac in Peru have provided the richest source of trepanated skulls. These skulls originate from several eras of prehistorical Inka culture about 3000 B. C. until Inka culture from the 10th until the 16th century A. D. [18, 109].

From the early interest shown in trepanation it can be surmised that cranioplasty must also have a long past. It went side by side through history with trepanation. It was not an unusual finding to see "Rondells" taken from other skulls and placed in trepanations of skulls deriving from European

Neolithicum. In old graves in Peru, gold and silver pieces have been found which corresponded to the skull defects in size and form. These can surely be considered a first attempt in cranioplasty [182].

In some primitive tribes of the Polynesian Islands, skull defects were repaired with coconut shell or even palm leaves and then covered with the scalp [137]. A number of scholars from the old world also discussed operations of cranial injuries. The first detailed description of an alloplastic closure of a

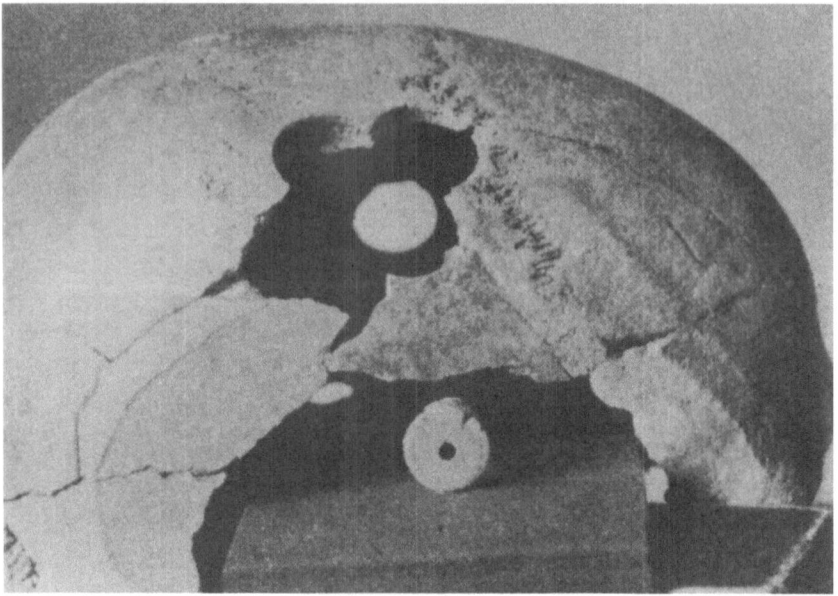

Fig. 2. A Celtic skull showing trepanation with a circular drill. "Rondells" (round discs) from another skull fitted into the burr holes

bone defect was not found before 1565. It was performed by Petronius, who used a gold plate for this purpose. 35 years later, in 1600, Fallopius recommended that noncontaminated bone with an intact dura be reimplanted into the trepanation. On the other hand, it was suggested that in skull defects caused by trauma it was better to remove the bone fragments and replace them with gold [137]. It is interesting to note that several contemporary doctors advised against using gold with the argument that this precious metal disappeared too often into the surgeon's pockets instead of serving to cover the skull defects.

In 1670, the Dutchman van Meekren performed a successful cranioplasty using canine bone. Opposition from the Church and the threat of excommunication led to the removal of the plastic [168].

From then on, till beyond the turn of the century, the closure of skull defects was looked upon as the classical domain in heteroplastics [107].

Schmidt (1893) used decalcified hare bone, Jaksch (1889) eagle bone, Rehn (1912) oxen horn, Henschen (1916) buffalo horn and Babock (1917) the cooked shoulder blade of a sheep ("the soupbone cranioplasty") [174].

There are still authors, in recent times, who have not given up using the heteroplastic method. For example, Haritonowa successfully covered a defect with a 2 mm thick piece of oxen horn in 1952. The heteroplastic method can indeed be successful when performed under optimal conditions in a closed bone area with no mechanical stress; in most cases, however, the material is rejected.

First reports of autoplastic cranical defect repair make mention of the following forms of trepanations: tibia with periosteum (Seydel), a skin-periosteum-bone flap (Wagner, Müller-König, Nicolladoni, von Hacker, Durante), a bone chip from the tabula externa (Keen 1905), rib with a double periosteum (Kappis 1905), shoulder blade with a double periosteum (Röpple 1912), as well as rib cartilage (Wilson 1918) [135, 154].

It was towards the end of the 19th century that celluloid was used as the first plastic material for cranioplasty [48]. Its alleged carcinogenic properties soon led to its being forgotten until plexiglass [93, 94] and a whole series of methylmethacrylates were developed from 1959 onwards. These acrylates (in particular Palacos® R)* proved to be non-irritable on the surrounding tissue.

A new era in reconstructive cranial surgery began in 1951, as Woringer published his method of cranioplasty with quick hardening acrylates, and Heppner put aside the earlier fears of cancer-stimulating acrylates [79]. Cranioplasty with methylacrylates has won first place in reconstructive cranial surgery thanks to its tissue compatibility and form stability.

---

* Schering Corporation U.S.A.

B. Clinical Aspects of Cranial Bone Defects

I. Origin of Cranial Defects

Defects in the skull bone can be either acquired or congenital [165, 169].

1. Acquired Defects

These are of various origin:

a) traumatic,
b) tumourous, i.e. caused by
   primary skull tumours (which originate in the skull bone or surroundings),
   secondary skull tumours (which originate from neighbouring, infiltrating
   tumours).

Moreover, they can result from:

c) bone infection (osteomyelitis),
d) decompressive trepanations.

Trauma is probably the most frequent cause of cranial defects, especially
there, where the bone is splittered or dirty. Usually, children or young people
are most affected.

Primary skull tumours, which may be the cause of skull defects, are mostly
different types of sarcomas (fibro-, osteo-, chondrosarcomas), osteomas and
chondromas as well as eosinophilic granulomas and cystic bone tumours [68,
169, 181].

Other tumours causing cranial defects by virtue of their progressive growth
are: dermoids and epidermoids, haemangiomas, reticulum cellsarcomas, Ewing
sarcomas.

Secondary bone tumours resulting in defects of the skull are: metastases,
meningiomas, dural epitheliomas (infiltrating) and tumours of the upper nasal
sinuses (neuroaesthesioblastomas) with infiltration of the fronto-basal region.

In our population of patients osteomas were identified in 3.2% of cases.
This incidence corresponds with reports in the literature [125, 172]. We found
no cases of osteosarcomas. Eosinophilic granulomas were diagnosed in 1.8%
of patients, which approximately corresponds to the frequency of such cases in

Zülch's collection of 6,000 tumours [55]. Bone cysts, haemangiomas and neoplastic deformities of the skull did not occur in our research period from 1969 until 1980. Intracranial tumours may also cause skull bone changes. Such a tumour can give rise to atrophy of the surrounding bone due to pressure and can force it out of its normal position or even infiltrate and completely destroy

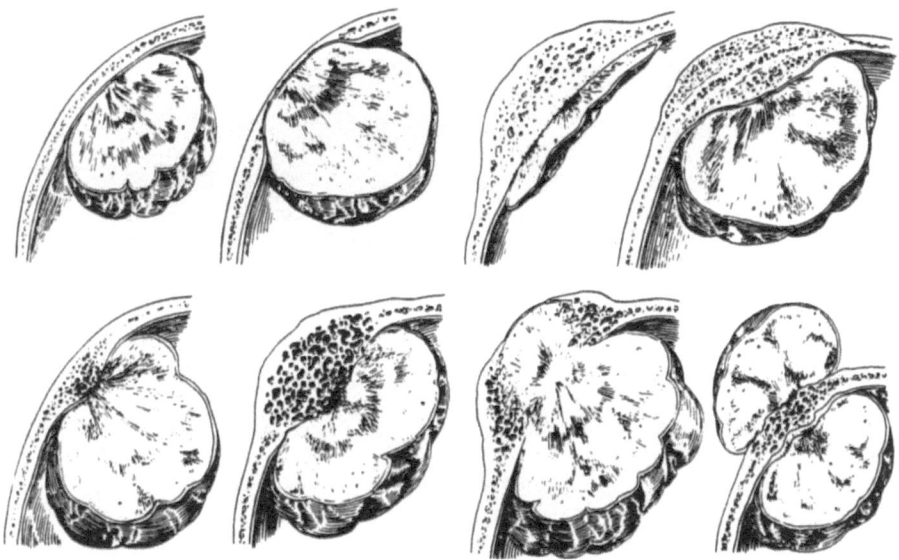

Fig. 3. Eight variations of meningioma growth and the resulting bone changes according to Cushing (from "Die zerebrale Angiographie" by H. Krayenbühl and M. G. Yaşargil. G. Thieme Verlag, Stuttgart 1956)

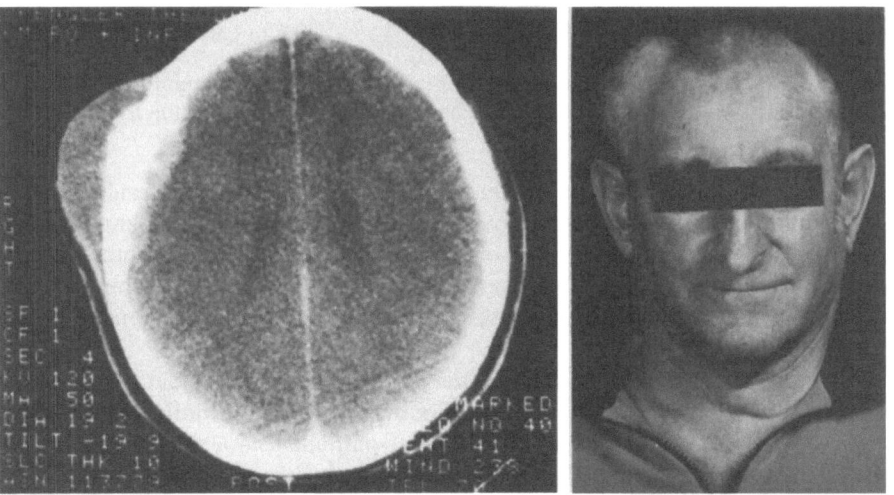

Fig. 4. Skull bone metastasis of a prostate carcinoma in a 61-year-old patient

it. This could particularly occur in the cases of meningiomas and bone
metastases. Among 217 treated cases with skull bone defects in our clinic 17%
were caused by intracranial tumours. Out of these, 13% were meningiomas
and 4% were due to metastases. The extensive statistics of Cushing,
Olivecrona and Zülch (see [55]) report meningiomas in 13–19%, metastases
in 3–5% and astrocytomas and glioblastomas in 20–45% of all brain
tumours [56, 125].

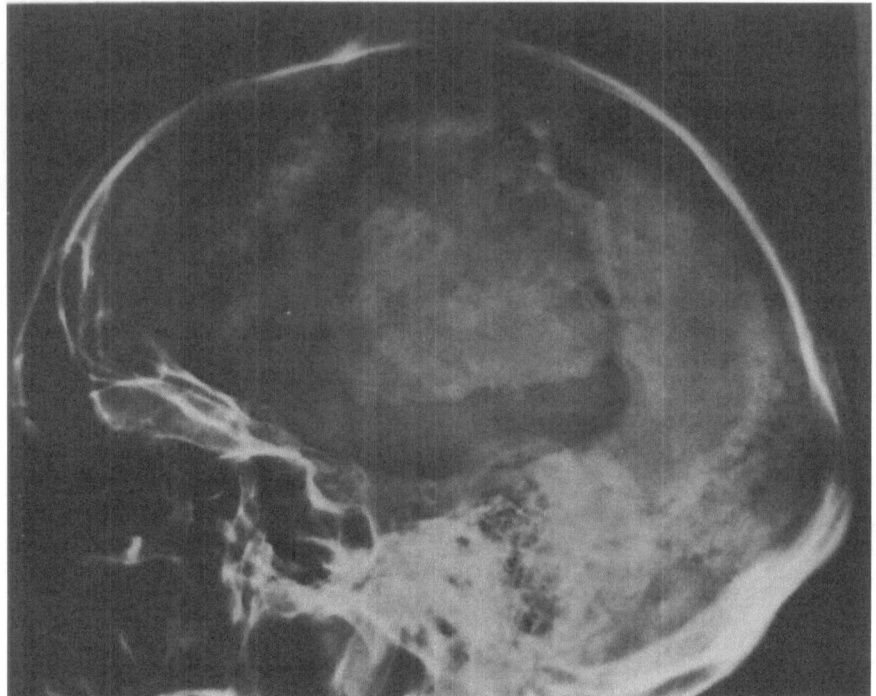

Fig. 5. A 48-year-old patient with osteomyelitis which developed 6 months after cranioplasty with his own bone; sequestration of bone pieces can be seen in the frontal region

Cranial osteomyelitis may develop after a latency period ranging from
several months to years. It is often found as a complication of a suppurative
process in the nasal sinuses (fronto-ethmoidal), after skull trepanation or open
brain injuries, and more seldom as a result of metastases. Apart from general
and local symptoms of inflammation, X-ray changes of the skull bone are also
evident [104].

As in practically all disorders of the skull bone, it is necessary to remove
completely the affected bone pieces. Treatment with antibiotics alone have
been of help in only a few cases. In 11 of our patients (5%), skull bone defects
were the result of osteomyelitis.

Before the introduction of urea and mannitol therapy, decompression
craniotomies were the only means to fight brain oedema. The introduction of

osmotherapy (urea, mannitol, corticosteroids) and especially barbiturate therapy, has drastically reduced the number of these operations in the last few years [23, 96]. Nevertheless, we performed decompressive trepanations in 27 (12.4%) patients in the period from 1969 until 1980. Cranial defects which are produced by decompressive trepanations in order to reduce effectively intracranial hypertension due to space occupying processes of various origins, form certainly a separate group of patients in which cranioplasty is indicated.

2. Congenital Defects

Congenital defects mostly result from dysraphic failures. In congenital skull defects symmetrical gaps in the bone can be found where the tabula interna is characteristically honey-comb-like and thinned (honey-comb skull), or where the bone is missing altogether (indented skull) [55]. The origin of these defects has not been understood. Such anomalies usually appear combined with other development disorders of the skeleton or central nervous organs. Claviculo-acromial dysostosis is an example where in addition to the skull bone defect the clavicula is not formed. We treated no such patients.

3. Demographic and Other Characteristics of Patients

In the Neurosurgical Clinic, Department of Surgery, University Hospital, Basel, altogether 217 patients of both sexes: 144 males (66%) and 73 females (34%) underwent cranioplasty during the period from 1969 to 1980. It is of interest to note that in 95 patients cranioplasty was performed with homologous bone bank: 84 with the patient's own and 11 with foreign bone. During this same period of time 122 skull defects were covered with acrylates. The age distribution of the patients is illustrated in Fig. 6. The youngest patient

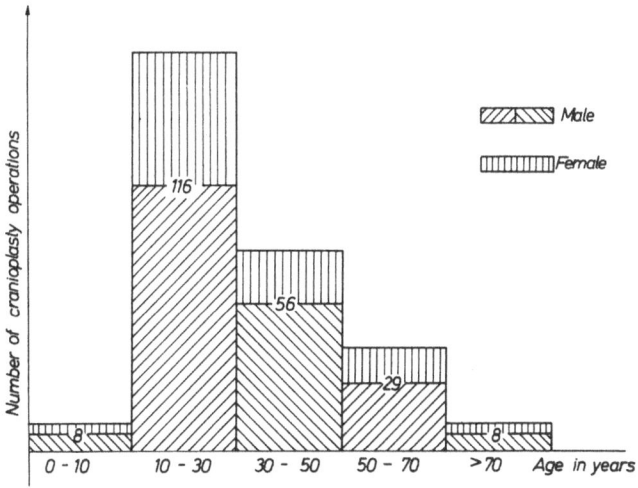

Fig. 6. Age distribution

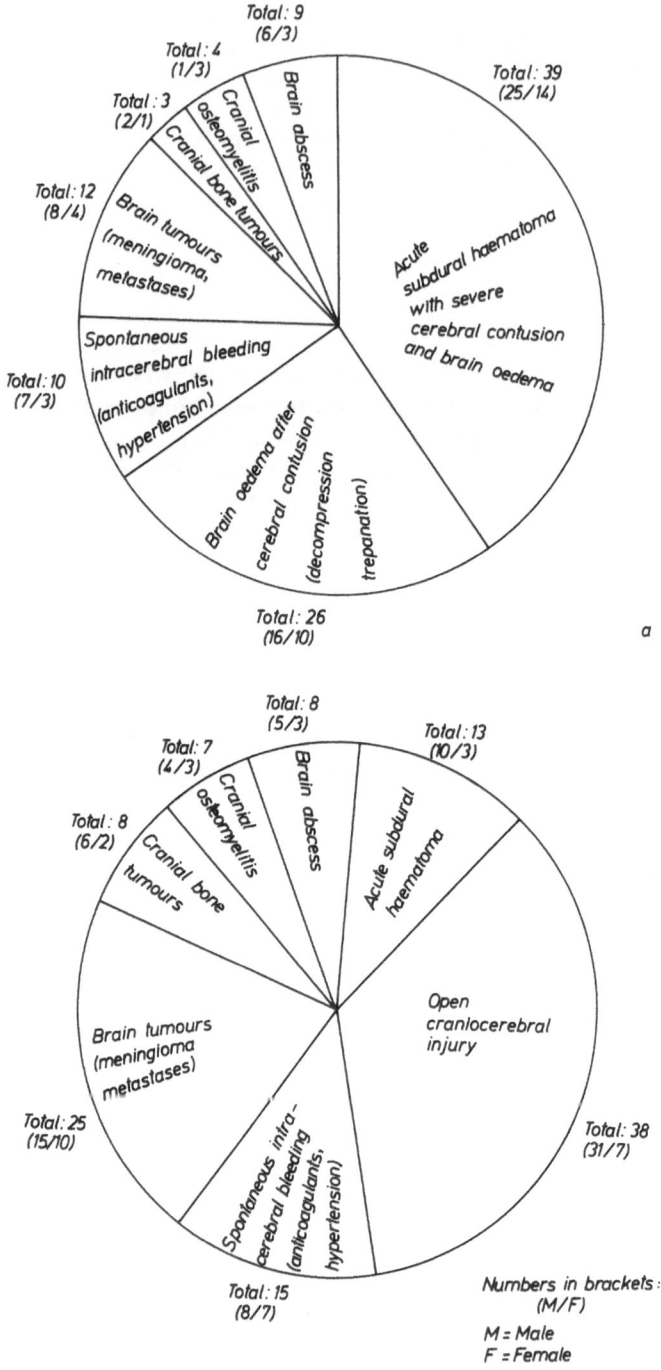

Total: 9
(6/3)

Total: 4
(1/3)

Total: 3
(2/1)

Total: 39
(25/14)

Total: 12
(8/4)

Cranial osteomyelitis

Cranial bone tumours

Brain abscess

Brain tumours (meningioma, metastases)

Spontaneous intracerebral bleeding (anticoagulants, hypertension)

Total: 10
(7/3)

Acute subdural haematoma with severe cerebral contusion and brain oedema

Brain oedema after cerebral contusion (decompression trepanation)

Total: 26
(16/10)

a

Total: 8
(5/3)

Total: 7
(4/3)

Total: 13
(10/3)

Total: 8
(6/2)

Cranial osteomyelitis

Cranial bone tumours

Brain abscess

Acute subdural haematoma

Brain tumours (meningioma metastases)

Open cranlocerebral injury

Total: 25
(15/10)

Spontaneous intra- cerebral bleeding (anticoagulants, hypertension)

Total: 38
(31/7)

Total: 15
(8/7)

Numbers in brackets: (M/F)

M = Male
F = Female

b

Fig. 7a. Diagram of the causes of cranial defects (103 patients, defects > 100 cm²)

Fig. 7b. Diagram of the causes of cranial defects (114 patients, defects < 100 cm²)

was 5 years and the oldest 78 years old. The highest percentage of cranioplasties falls into the age group of 10–30 years (53%). This appears to be the
high-risk population group also in terms of the rate of accidents leading to
severe head injuries. Second ranking is the age group of 30–50 years. There
was no difference in the number of cranioplasties performed in the youngest
and in the oldest age groups, which were represented with 8 patients each.
With regard to sex and age we found no notable difference in the
postoperative recovery and wound healing after cranioplasty.

Craniocerebral injuries appear to be the most frequent primary event
leading to the skull defects. In 53.4% of our patients head injuries with various
deleterious primary and secondary consequences preceded cranioplasty
(Figs. 7 a, b).

Brain tumours were also represented in a considerable proportion of our
patients. Interestingly, whereas in respect to the latter cause no sex differences
were apparent, there was a marked prevalence of males in craniocerebral
injury groups.

Large bone defects of more than 100 cm² were present in 103 (47.5%) and
small ones of less than 100 cm² in 114 (52.5%) patients. Large cranial defects
were more often due to secondary consequences of head injuries than the
small ones.

II. Neurological and Psychic Changes Before and After Cranioplasty

Large decompression craniotomies are often a life saving procedure in
patients where a massive cerebral oedema does not respond to conservative
methods [96]. A few months after a decompression craniotomy the taunt skin
flap begins to sink and neurological and psychic changes then appear [162]. A
lack of appropriate methods to investigate these changes was the reason why
they have not been understood or described in a more detailed way. The
causes were first looked for in degenerative changes, CSF (cerebrospinal fluid)
circulation disturbances and cerebral blood flow disturbances. Even in the
1950's it was rare that neuroradiology (carotis angiogram, pneumo-encephalo-
gram) was used to investigate this problem. Apart from cases with obvious
brain mass displacement, these aggressive methods only rarely helped in
analyzing the factors responsible for neurological and psychic changes due to
cranial defects.

Furthermore, the surgical repairing methods were not even considered as
possible therapeutic measure. Not so long ago, in 1948, Grantham and Landis
argued, after analyzing 100 cases of large decompression craniotomies, that the
major value of cranioplasty was the repair of the cosmetic defect [66].
Although they were impressed by the fact that nearly all patients of this group
with aphasia showed marked improvements of their speech difficulties after
cranioplasty, they denied a relationship between these changes and the
operation.

2*

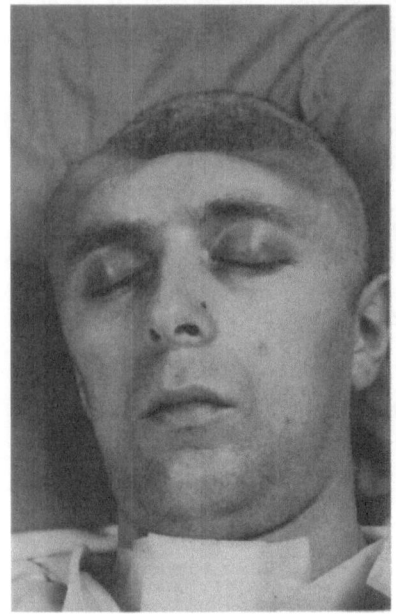 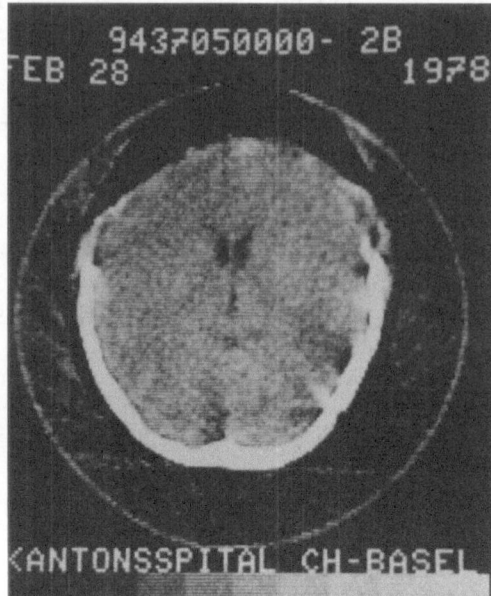

Fig. 8a   Fig. 8b

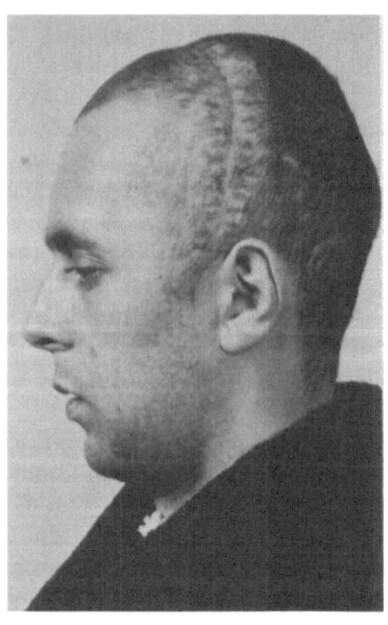 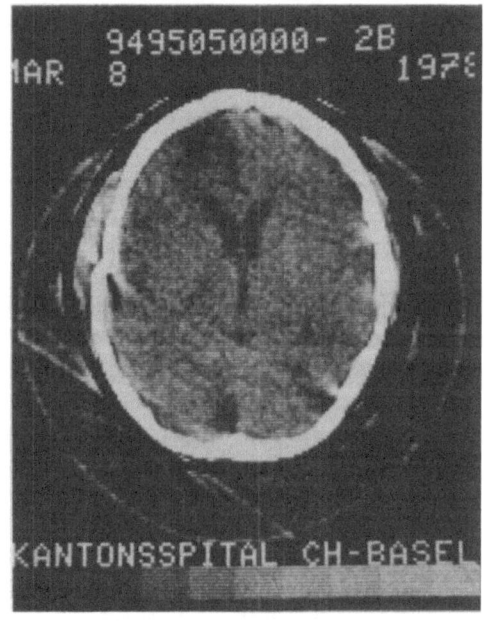

Fig. 9a   Fig. 9b

Of interest is a report showing that in a patient one year after closure of the cranial defect, dramatic improvement of the neurological disturbances was evident [66]. The main reason for that was, however, not recognized, although it was supposed that the improvement was of intracranial origin and that the concave, flaccid skin flap represented only an external manifestation of the intracranial changes. This phenomenon, however, was not further investigated.

The introduction of computerized tomography (CT) in 1974 marks in this respect a turning point [159]. This method is easily applied, generally without risk, regardless of the age and condition of the patient. The CT revealed remarkable intracranial changes which may follow craniotomies. For example, an advanced hemisphere deformation as well as marked brain mass displacement and ventricle deformation is illustrated in Fig. 8b. The assumption that pathological intracranial changes are intimately related to neurological and psychic changes has been further supported by such observations [162, 186].

1. Classification of Neurological Deficits and of the Skin Flap Types

In the course of events, patients with larger cranial defects may develop various neurological and psychic symptoms which are unrelated to the primary pathology causing the defect. The most commonly observed symptoms are headaches, dizziness, vertigo, general discomfort, irritability, different degrees of cognitive disturbances, dysphasia, paresis of extremities and others. Epileptic fits may also occur.

According to the severity of the neurological and psychic impairment, we have categorized the patients into four groups:

0 = normal neurological status without psychic changes;

1 = minimal neurological deficit with discrete hemi- or monoparesis, some difficulty finding words and slight psychoorganic disturbances;

2 = moderate neurological deficit with hemi- or monoparesis but without marked disability of the patient, dysphasia, however, allowing certain degree of communication, and psychoorganic syndrome with preserved orientation;

3 = severe neurological deficit with hemiparalysis, complete aphasia, mostly without sphincter control, and severe psychoorganic changes. All these patients are reliant on outside help.

Fig. 8a. A 27-year-old patient with a bone flap decompression on both sides, 3 weeks after the removal of an acute subdural haematoma. Marked sinking-in of the wound, severe psychoorganic syndrome with somnolence (patient only slightly reacting)

Fig. 8b. CT shows a distinct compression of the anterior regions of both brain hemispheres with ventricle deformation

Fig. 9a. The same patient as in Fig. 8a, 3 weeks after cranioplasty. Visible improvement in the psychoorganic syndrome and level of consciousness

Fig. 9b. CT: Normalization of the intracranial state

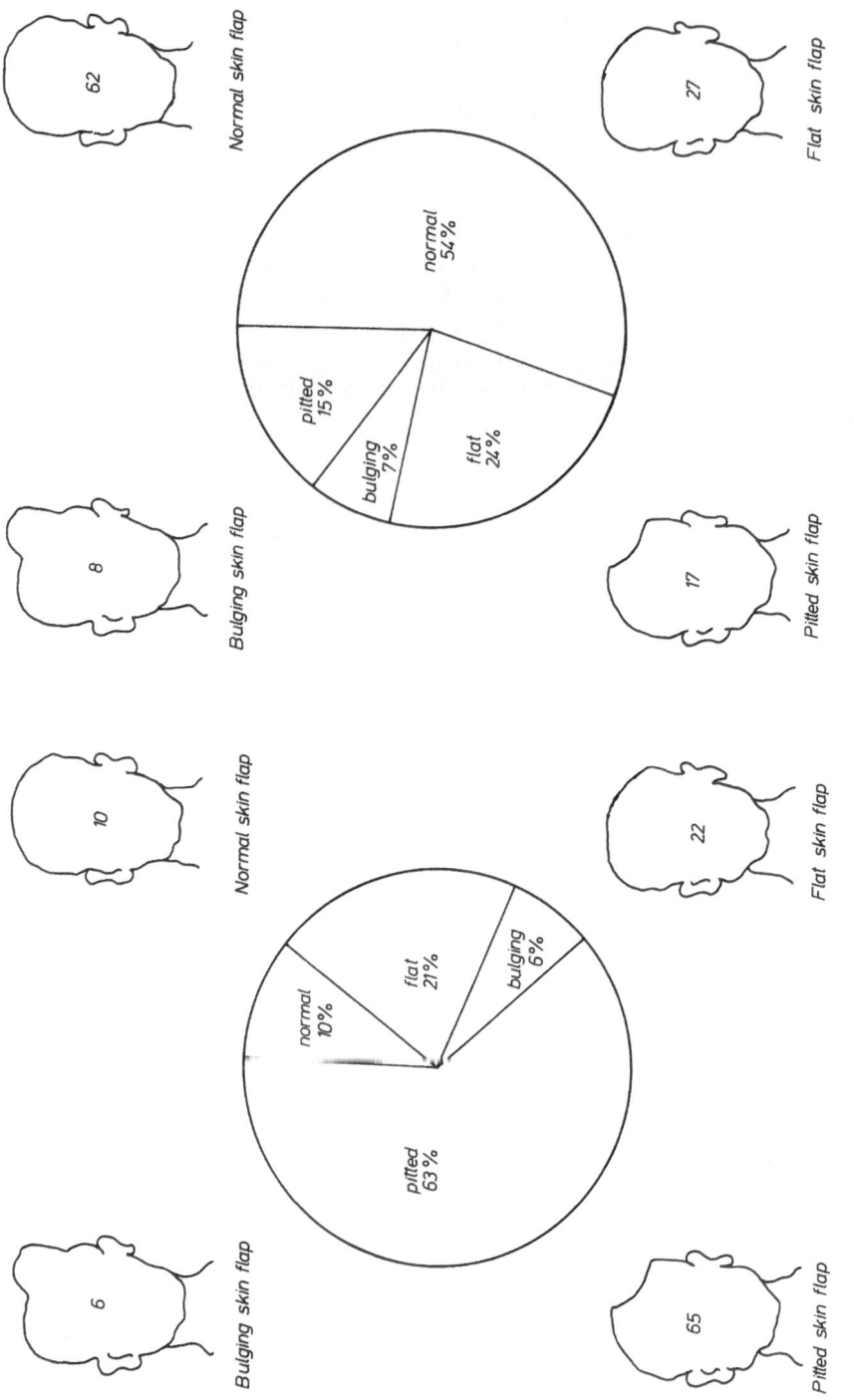

Fig. 10b. Skin flap status: 114 patients with a cranial bone defect smaller than 100 cm²

Fig. 10a. Skin flap status: 103 patients with a cranial bone defect of over 100 cm²

The configuration of the skin flap is an important factor in determining the severity of the neurological symptoms. Based upon the configuration of the skin flap in the standing position, four types of skin flaps could be discriminated:

a) concave, flaccid (sunken-in) skin flap,
b) flat skin flap,
c) normal, convex skin flap,
d) bulging skin flap.

A predisposing factor for the formation of concave, sunken-in skin flap are cranial defects with surface larger than 100 cm². We found such skin flaps in 63% of all patients with large skull defects. Normal skin flap configuration in such patients was found only in 9.7% of cases (10 patients). Different configurations of skin flaps and their distribution among the patients with skull defects larger than 100 cm² are illustrated in Fig. 10 (a, b).

Normal skin flap dominated in patients with smaller cranial defects. We found it in 54% of our patients with cranial defects of less than 100 cm². In 15% of such patients, however, concave, flaccid skin flap was also found.

Severe neurological and psychic symptoms were observed exclusively in patients with large and sunken-in skin flap (Tables 1 and 2). Among altogether

Table 1. *103 Patients, Defect >100 cm²*

Neurological status	Skin flap status				
	Normal	Flat	Bulging	Pitted	Total
Normal	6	15	1	12	34
Minimal neurological symptoms	4	2	1	14	21
Neurological symptoms of a moderate degree	–	5	4	17	26
Severe neurological symptoms	–	–	–	22	22
Total	10	22	6	65	103

Table 2. *114 Patients, Defect <100 cm²*

Neurological status	Skin flap status				
	Normal	Flat	Bulging	Pitted	Total
Normal	51	17	2	7	77
Minimal neurological symptoms	8	8	4	4	24
Neurological symptoms of a moderate degree	3	2	2	6	13
Severe neurological symptoms	–	–	–	–	–
Total	62	27	8	17	114

103 patients with large skull defects 33% showed, however, no neurological impairment, whereas minimal or moderate disturbances were diagnosed in 20 and 25% respectively.

In the majority of patients with smaller skull defects and normal skin flap neurological symptoms were absent (67%) or minimal.

As already mentioned, besides the size of the skull defects, its configuration is very much determining the clinical picture of the patients. Whereas the size of the defect is directly proportional to the extent of the primary injury or pathology, the skin flap is, by contrast, an indirect sign of the extent of intracranial, secondary changes.

2. The "Sinking Skin Flap Syndrome"

In a certain proportion of patients with large cranial defects, considerable displacement of the brain, combined with deformation of the ventricles and, finally, brain collapse, develops weeks or months after an extensive craniotomy [161, 162]. These changes are unrelated to the primary cause of the skull bone defect. Upon examination, strongly pitted wound and heavily retracted skin flap are found in such patients. In addition, the majority of them (see before) exhibits disabling clinical, neurological as well as psychic symptoms. Some of these symptoms are aggravated by changes of the posture of the body. The clinical syndrome accompanying heavily retracted, concave, sunken-in skin flap has been described by numerous authors as „syndrome of the trephined", the "postconcussive or posttraumatic syndrome", and by japanese authors in 1977 [186] as "syndrome of the sinking skin flap" (Figs. 11a, b).

The cause of the sinking skin flap syndrome has not been entirely explained. Among various factors suggested to be causally related to the development of this syndrome, the difference between the intracranial and atmospheric pressure has been particularly emphasized [156, 162, 186]. It was suggested that as a consequence of this condition, the cerebrospinal fluid is pressed out of the skull cavity, which results in the reduction of its intracranial volume ([39, 40, 47], for further details see also later).

The following example refers to the notion that atmospheric pressure is an essential factor influencing the intracranial contents of an uncovered skull: brain prolapse occurred in patients with open craniocerebral injuries when they were transported by air at a high altitude. This complication was avoided by the transport in modern planes, with hermetically insulated cabins and a controlled atmospheric pressure (pressurized cabins) [124].

The increase in the volume of the brain was supposed to be caused by several factors: firstly, through the spread of air infiltrating into the inner subarachnoid space and secondly, through the rise in pressure of the CSF caused by a decrease in the atmospheric pressure and an increase in vascular filling as a result of oxygen deficiency [124].

We have observed 10 patients with sinking skin flap syndrome where the total surface of skull defects was larger than 100 cm². In all patients CT identified brain mass displacement with brain collapse and ventricle deformation. In 8 patients, the syndrome developed after large bone flap decompression craniotomies, performed because of the brain oedema, following the removal of a large acute subdural haematoma. One skull defect resulted from the removal of a convexity meningioma with cranial bone infiltration. In another patient there was a large, spontaneous intracerebral haematoma due to untreated hypertension. The youngest patient was 18 years and the oldest 72 years old. The cranioplasty preparations, particularly created to cover the existing large defects, as well as the surgical intervention itself, took a normal course in all patients. There were practically no complications, apart from a temporary tachycardia in a few patients. The CT examinations which were repeated immediately after the cranioplasty showed the full expansion of the brain.

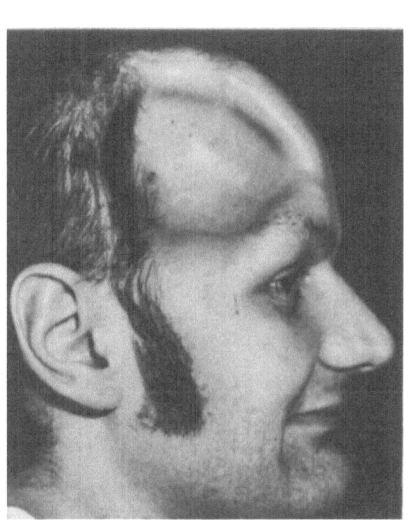
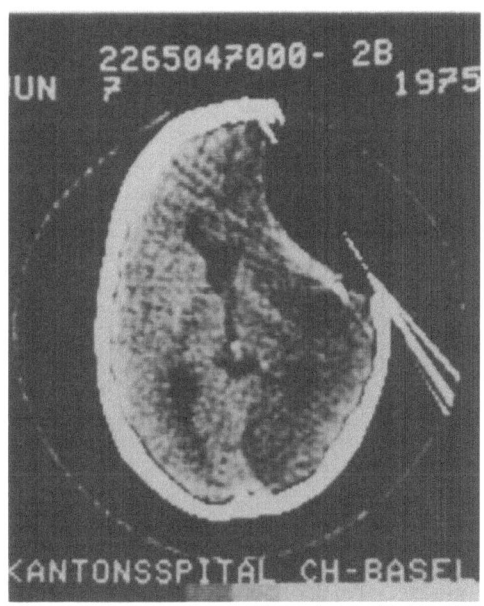

Fig. 11 a   Fig. 11 b

Fig. 11a. A 35-year-old patient with bone flap decompression, 6 months after the removal of an acute subdural haematoma. Obvious "Sinking Skin Flap Syndrome"

Fig. 11b. CT of the skull: severe intracranial changes (brain mass displacement, cerebral compression, ventricle deformation), accompanied by a left, spastic hemiplegia and POS

3. The Influence of Cranioplasty Upon Neurological and Psychic Changes

From a total of 217 patients postoperative control was done in 170 (78%). In examinations carried out between 6 months and 2 years after the intervention, 81 patients (78.6%) of altogether 103 patients with large bone

Table 3. *Postoperative Control of Patients with Large Skull Defects (>100 cm²)*

Degree of change	Neurological symptoms	Partial improvement after cranioplasty	Complete improvement after cranioplasty	Unchanged after cranioplasty	Not controlled	Died	Total
	Normal neurological condition	–	–	28	6	–	34
Minimal	Discrete hemiplegia	2	7	3	–	–	12
Minimal	Speech and memory disturbances	1	2	–	–	–	3
Minimal	Slight psychic changes with headache, dizziness etc.	3	2	1	–	–	6
Moderate	Hemiparesis	4	4	2	1	2	13
Moderate	Speech disturbances	1	1	–	–	–	2
Moderate	Psychorganic syndrome (POS)	2	–	1	–	1	4
Moderate	Dizziness, headaches, ataxia, balance disorder	2	4	1	–	–	7
	Total	15	20	36	7	3	81

defects were controlled. Of these, 69 patients had preoperatively neurological symptoms of various degrees of intensity. 10 patients had died and 12 did not appear for the check-up. The Tables 3 and 4 illustrate the recovery rate in the patients of this group.

In the group of patients with small skull defects, 89 (78%) out of 114 patients were controlled: 60 of them were patients with a normal preoperative neurological status. Table 5 summarizes the postoperative control findings in this group. It is to be mentioned that in this group we did not observe any patient with severe neurological symptoms. In 20 (49%) patients (both from the group with large and small defects) with minimal deficits we observed a complete disappearance of the symptoms. In these patients, flat and normal skin flap configuration predominated. In the patients with moderate neurological deficiencies we could verify a complete recovery in 11 cases (35%) of the 31 controlled.

Table 4. *Postoperative Control of Patients with Severe Preoperative Neurological Symptoms and Large Skull Defects*

Neurological symptoms	Partial improvement after cranioplasty	Complete improvement after cranioplasty	Unchanged after cranioplasty	Not controlled	Died	Total
Hemiparesis with aphasia	3	1	1	4	2	11
Severe POS and hemiparesis	2	–	1	–	3	6
Aphasia, dizziness, headaches, ataxia	–	1	1	1	2	5
Total	5	2	3	5	7	22

Table 5. *Postoperative Control of Patients with Small Defects of the Skull*

Degree of change	Neurological symptoms	Partial improvement after cranioplasty	Complete improvement after cranioplasty	Unchanged after cranioplasty	Not controlled	Died	Total
	Normal neurological condition	–	–	60	15	2	77
Minimal	Discrete hemiplegia	1	4	2	2	–	9
	Speech and memory disturbances	2	1	1	–	–	4
	Slight psychic changes, headache, dizziness, others	3	4	2	2	–	11
Moderate	Hemiparesis	2	1	–	1	–	4
	Speech disturbances	1	–	–	1	–	2
	POS, hemiparesis	1	–	1	–	1	3
	Dizziness, headache, ataxia	2	1	–	1	–	4
	Total	12	11	60	22	3	114

Our experiences show that patients with minimal neurological symptoms and with normal or flat skin flaps have the best chance of recovery: 44% of these patients showed complete recovery after the operation. Second-best prognosis have patients with neurological and psychic changes of a moderate degree. Nevertheless, we have observed here a complete recovery in 11 out of the 39 controlled patients. Of the 22 patients with severe neurological symptoms, 12 (54.5%) were not accessible for a check-up in the course of the postoperative period. This number undoubtedly speaks for the grave fate of these patients. We observed here only 2 complete recoveries after cranioplasty

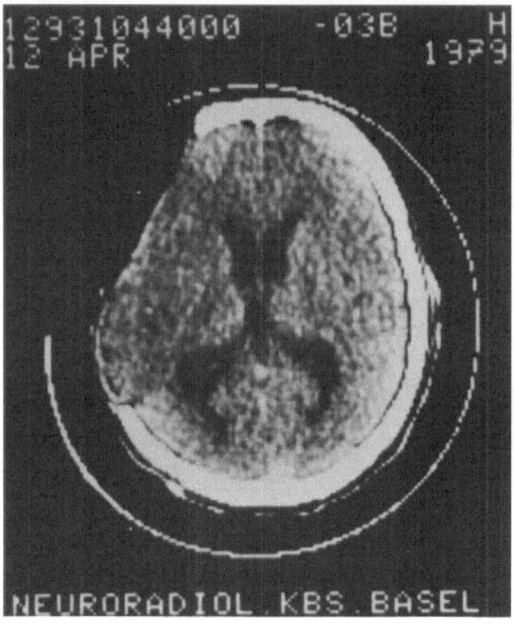

Fig. 12. Large skull defect with pitted skin flap and slight hemisphere compression. Neither brain mass displacement nor ventricle deformation are present. No neurological symptoms

(9%), 5 patients showed partial improvement and 3 further patients remained in the same condition. Realising how seriously handicapped and disabled the patients of this group are, the result that besides 2 full recoveries about 23% of the patients recovered at least partially, must be considered as satisfactory.

In view of previous experiences, it appears unusual and surprising that in 34 (33%) of 103 patients with skull defects larger than 100 cm² no neurological symptoms were found. The explanation may possibly be that, as shown in Fig. 12, in fact no displacement of the brain mass developed in these patients. A slight hemisphere deformation and a ventricle collapse were apparently still within the range of the adaptation capabilities of the brain.

III. Electroencephalographic (EEG) Changes in Patients with Cranial Defects

The pathophysiological mechanisms underlying epileptic disorders are still not understood. This is also true for posttraumatic or residual epilepsies, which develop in a certain number of patients after head injuries and craniotomies. In the first half of this century rather widespread was the hypothesis that these types of epilepsy result from the "scar tension" produced by adhesions between the skin, dura and the brain surface [33, 65, 111]. Based on this assumption, the term "scar epilepsy" was generated to define this type of epilepsy [33, 38, 99, 187].

It is of interest to note that in order to prevent the renewed formation of cicatrice after cranioplasty and supposed seizure-eliciting movements of skin flaps on unclosed cranial defect, implantation of fat into the cavity resulting from scar removal was sometimes performed [33, 111]. However, this method has proved unsuccessful not only because of the high risk of infection, but also because it failed to serve the purpose.

As a treatment of choice in posttraumatic seizures, early cranioplasty was emphasized by many authors in the past. In 1939 Grant, for instance, reported the decrease in the incidence and even complete disappearance of epileptic fits in 18 out of 27 patients (67%) in which cranioplasty was performed. Several other authors described similar findings, however, mostly in small numbers of patients [38, 53, 54, 65, 99, 136]. The improvements observed after cranioplasty were attributed to the removal of adhesions between the skin and the dura [63]. Controversial views, however, about the benefit of cranial repair in posttraumatic epilepsy, have appeared later on, in particular after World War II [177].

Erculei and Walker [43], reviewing the postoperative course in a rather large population of patients, found no conclusive evidence that cranial repair exerts determining influence on posttraumatic epilepsy. Such doubts were also raised by other authors arguing that nearly always only cranial defect is repaired, while the brain cicatrice and the adhesions between the dura and the brain surface remain [111, 177]. Therefore, the "scar tension" could further exert its effects. If in spite of that the patients show reduced incidence of seizures, the reason for that was assumed to be another, independent factor. Along this line, the repairing surgery seemed to be justified only if cortical "epilepsy resection" could be performed. Additional postulated requirements for cranioplasty were the restoration of physiological proportions of the brain within the brain cavity besides the removal of scars and adhesions [43, 111].

The existing controversies and the fact that not too many studies about clinical and electroencephalographic changes in epileptic patients undergoing cranioplasty have been reported until now [111, 123, 187], have stimulated our interest in this problem.

1. EEG Recordings and Casuistic

EEG examinations were performed before and after cranioplasty in altogether 20 patients with cranial defects larger than 100 cm². The recordings were taken, with one exception, between 2 weeks and 1 day before, and between 1 week and 6 months after the repair of the defect. One patient was controlled also 10 months after surgery.

Usual criteria for EEG changes were applied [76]:

a) general changes in the curve shapes,
b) presence or absence of sub-delta-theta focus and
c) presence or absence of epileptic potential (spikes and sharp waves).

Cranioplasty operations were carried out between 3 months and 4 years after craniotomy. The youngest patient was 21 and the oldest 70 years old. 12 cranioplasty operations were performed with acrylate (Palacos® R with Gentamycin®) and 8 patients received a closure with their own bone, which had been stored in the bone bank after a decompression craniotomy. Half of the patients (10) had serious brain injuries (included was one suicide attempt with gun-shot wounds) with acute subdural haematomas, where an intraoperative brain oedema developed and, therefore, a bone decompression had to be undertaken. In 4 patients (3 convexity and 1 parasagittal meningioma) the skull defect was due to bone destruction caused by tumour infiltration. In 4 patients operated for vascular deformities (3 basal aneurysms and 1 occipital AV-fistula), skull defect resulted because of infection (n = 2) and because of intraoperative brain oedema (n = 2). In one case of an intra-cerebral haematoma with hypertension and brain abscess, the skull bone was removed because of the acute development of brain swelling.

2. Evaluation of EEG Changes

Of 20 examined patients, 6 (3%) suffered preoperatively of grand-mal type epileptic seizures. Epilepsy was of various duration as well as varying intensity and seizures frequency. In the remaining 12 patients, pathological EEG recordings were not accompanied by overt epileptic fits.

Of 4 patients from whom we removed a meningioma and all of whom had grand-mal epilepsy preoperatively, 2 cases showed electroencephalographic improvement postoperatively, in one EEG there were no changes and another one showed deterioration in the findings. The deterioration was due to a recurrent, malignant meningioma, the patient had to be operated again and died shortly afterwards.

In 5 of 10 patients with craniocerebral injuries (acute subdural haematomas), we found considerably improved EEG in all 3 criteria. In 3 cases the EEG after cranioplasty remained unchanged, and of the 2 cases which showed considerable deterioration, one patient (66 years old) did not recover from the operation and, as a matter of fact, died a few months later from aspiration pneumonia.

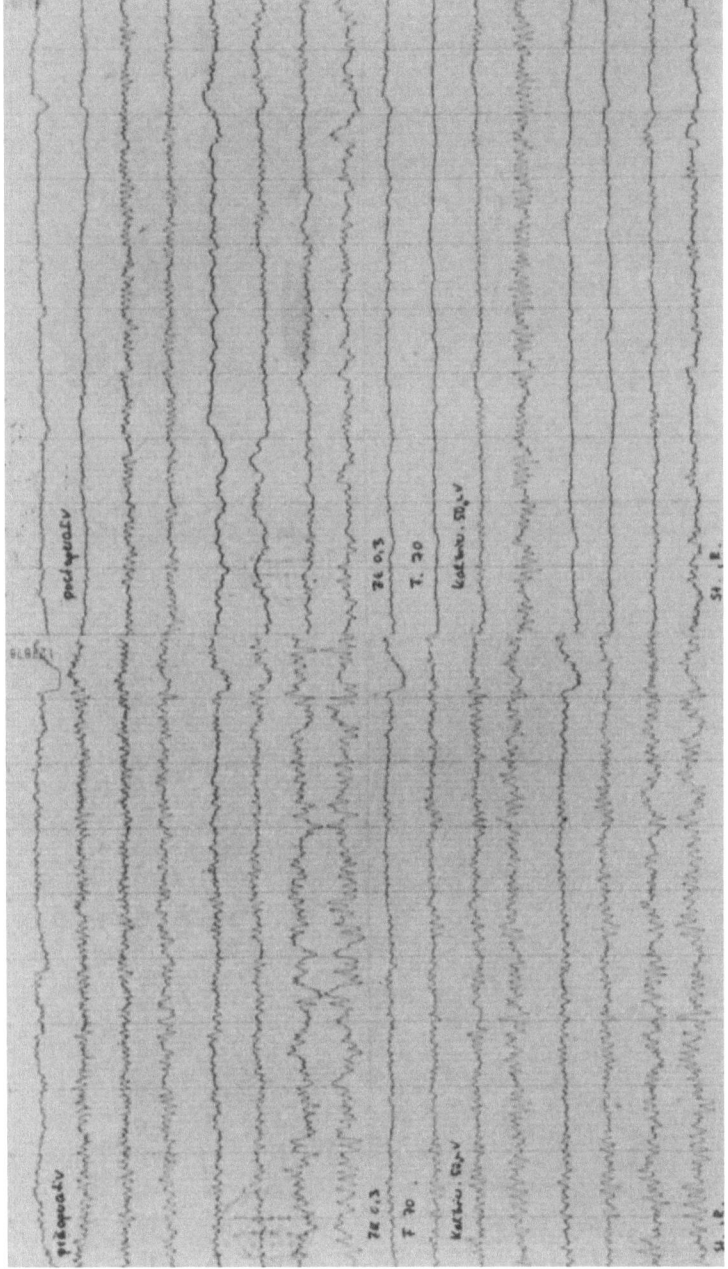

Fig. 13. Visible improvement in the EEG curve after cranioplasty in a patient with an operated brain abscess

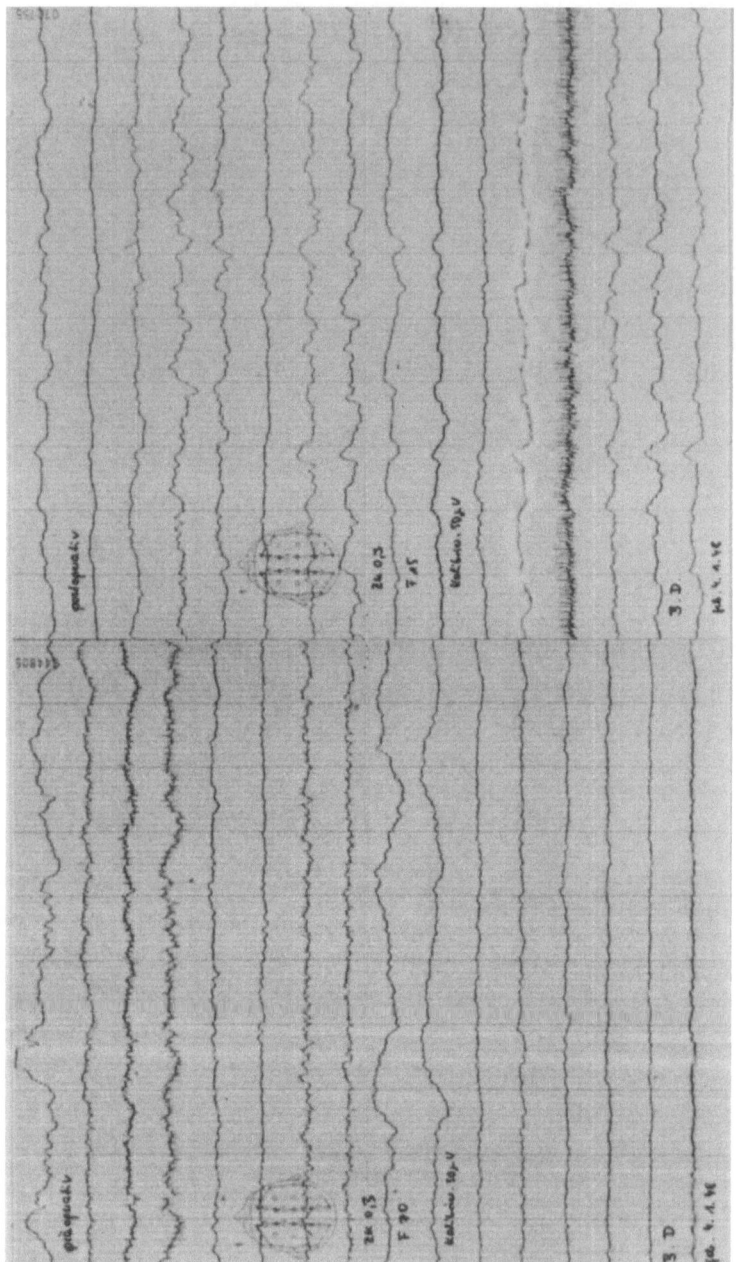

Fig. 14. Deterioration of the EEG curve after cranioplasty and drainage of a spontaneous intracerebral haematoma in a patient with hypertension

Of 4 patients with operated vascular deformities (3 basal aneurysms and 1 AV-fistula) general improvement was verified in 3 cases in which the pre-existing focal disturbances disappeared. In the remaining case, however, the EEG curve did not show any marked change after the cranioplasty. In another patient, operated for brain abscess in the left temporal region, considerable improvement of the EEG was seen after cranioplasty. The pre- and postoperative EEG findings are illustrated in Fig. 13.

As seen in Fig. 13 "sharp waves" and "spikes" have disappeared and focal disturbances were not visible. Therefore, a general postoperative stabilisation of the EEG findings could be demonstrated. Fig. 14, by contrast, illustrates deterioration in the EEG findings, which was observed after cranioplasty in a patient with hypertension and a spontaneous intracerebral haematoma in the basal ganglia region.

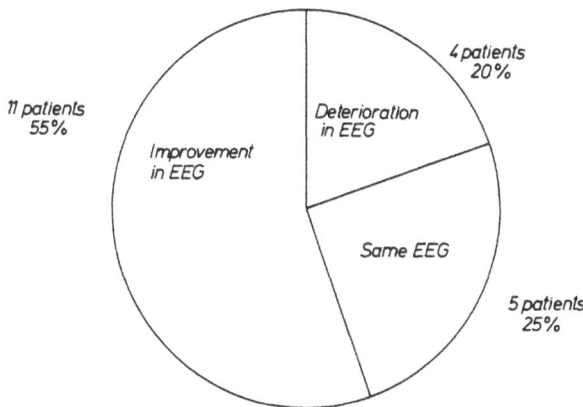

Fig. 15. Diagram of EEG findings in 20 patients after cranioplasty

From all EEG-recordings, unchanged findings in comparison with the preoperative status were found in altogether 5 patients (25%). In fact, also no clinical improvement was found in these cases. In 4 (20%) patients general deterioration of the EEG was diagnosed. Of these 4 patients, 2 did not recover and died in the further course of the illness (1 from aspiration pneumonia and 1 from recurrent malignant meningioma). The immediate postoperative EEG deterioration of the other 2 patients could not be explained, as these patients showed satisfactory and uneventful clinical recovery. However, it should be stressed that in both cases the EEG was taken quite early: after the 5th and 7th day after cranioplasty. The patients were discharged from hospital thereafter and did not present themselves for further control.

Fig. 15 summarizes the observations related to global EEG findings in our patient population. It is noteworthy that of 6 patients with grand-mal epileptic seizures, five patients remarkably improved in that in 3 of them the seizures recurred only sporadically, and in 2 others the seizures did not appear at all during the whole postoperative observation period (6 months). In one case no improvement was observed.

Although the experience based on observation of 20 cases is certainly limited, results up to now support the notion that cranioplasty has a positive effect on the EEG findings as well as on the improvement of epilepsy. The fact that in 11 (55%) patients the pre-existing pathological EEG obviously improved and that the cranioplasty had a clear-cut beneficial effect in 5 out of 6 patients with preoperative epileptic seizures, is an encouraging finding. In this respect, the repairing and therapeutic benefit of cranioplasty should not be underestimated.

IV. Scintigraphy Findings in Patients with Cranial Bone Defects

Scintigraphy of cranioplasty was first carried out at the beginning of 1970. The application of this method was stimulated by the discovery of grey, glassy-spongy, highly vascularized granulation tissue, which developed under the plastic implant in the epidural space [101]. The scintigraphic examinations were, however, limited to the postoperative stage and were uniquely performed in cranioplasty with acrylates. Since the picture obtained was interpreted as a sign of irritation, brain scintigraphy appeared to be an excellent method to examine the extent of the formation of granulation and the reaction of the surrounding tissue to methylmethacrylate. The spread of granulation tissue served as a criterion of the irritation potential of the prosthesis material.

The scintigraphic changes which were found displayed a calotte-shaped distribution of increased activity of radionuclides below the cranioplasty. Of 14 patients with acrylate closures, examined at that time, in 5 the scintigraphy was done with technetium 99-M-pertechnate and in 9 with strontium 87-M-citrate. The examinations were performed between 4 months and 7 years postoperatively. The deposition of the different radionuclides, which in 70% of the patients was found underneath as well as on the top of the acrylate implant, was identified pathohistologically as a non-specific granulation tissue [101].

After a single intravenous dose of 10–15 mCi 99mTc pertechnate or Tc-gluconeptomate, the perfusion was examined with the "dynamic" vascular scintigram in intervals of 1–5 seconds. Thereby, the state of blood flow in the neck, skull and cerebral arteries, their capillary ramification as well as the venous return could be followed up. Also, a right to left comparison could be performed with the help of computer analysis. Further, by the conventional "statical" scintigram the integrity of the blood-brain barrier in the dispersion area of the carotis interna as well as the cranial area encompassing the carotis externa could be identified [51].

Moreover, changes in the intracranial structures, for example hemisphere movements and the condition of epi- and subdural spaces in the vicinity of the cranioplasty could be examined by this method [188].

Computer tomographical examinations of the intracranial contents in patients with cranial defects, which we have systematically carried out for the first time [159], have revealed very unusual and so far partly unknown changes. Large hemisphere and ventricle deformations on the side of the uncovered skull and marked brain mass displacements on the contra-lateral side, sometimes accompanied by described severe neurological and psychic

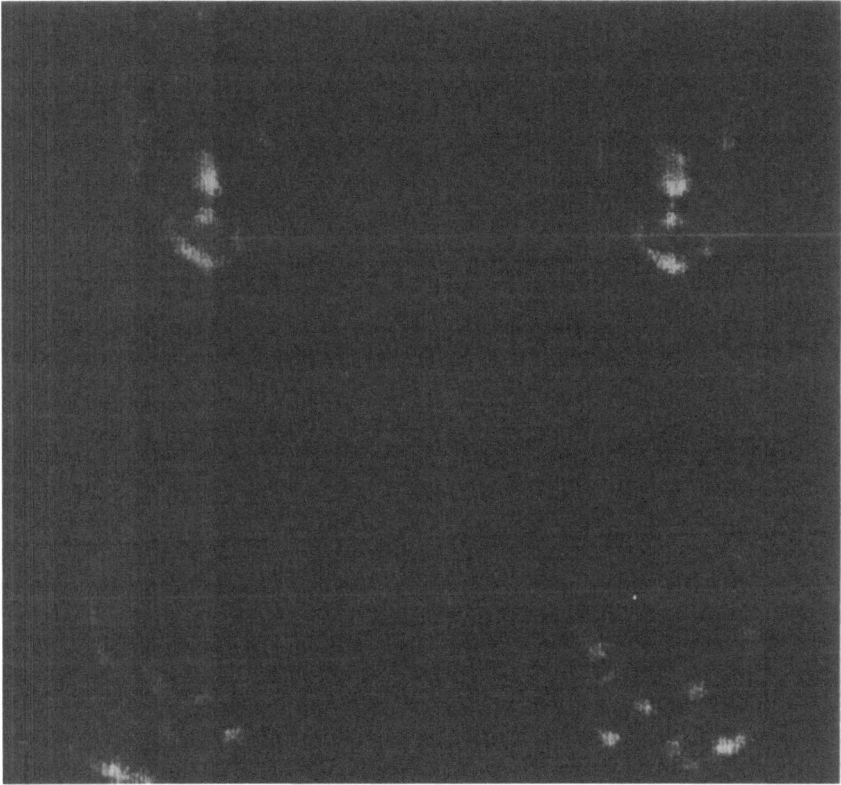

Fig. 16. A 53-year-old patient after removal of a right parieto-temporal intracerebral haematoma. Marked accumulation of radionuclides in the pitted wound area with slight displacement of the midline towards the left

symptoms [162], were discovered. In our opinion as well as in other authors', under such massive pathological conditions, circulation and perfusion of the brain must also be abnormal [14]. In view of this, scintigraphic investigations in cranial defects seemed warranted. The brain segments lying under the cranio-plasty and the contact sites between cranioplasty and skull where often – as a response to irritation – an increased osseous reconstruction or formation takes place [32, 35, 156], were also examined by scintigraphy.

1. Casuistic

The object of our study were 10 patients (3 females and 7 males); the youngest was 29 and the oldest 65 years old. Brain meningiomas were removed from 2 patients, 1 female patient had a spontaneous intracerebral bleeding caused by hypertension, and in 1 patient the skull defect was the result of a wound infection after the removal of an AV-fistula. The 6 other patients had severe craniocerebral injuries with acute subdural haematomas; a bone flap decompression had to be performed because of brain oedema which developed during the operation and remained uninfluenced by drugs. In 4 cases the cranioplasty was performed with acrylate (Palacos® R with Gentamycin®), and in 6 cases with the patient's own bone. All scintigraphical examinations of the brain were carried out under identical conditions before and after the skull closure in each patient. The examination time was on the average 3 days before the closure and 3 weeks postoperatively. Before cranioplasty, a brain mass displacement with an accumulation of the radionuclides in the pitted wound area was detected in 7 patients by conventional scintigraphy.

2. Results and Discussion

Scintigraphically, no brain mass displacement was detected in 3 patients with smaller bone defects and a less pitted wound area; however, although the concentration of radionuclides in the skull defect area was not too intense, it was visibly increased by comparison to normality. In these patients the "dynamic" scintigram showed normal symmetrical brain hemisphere perfusion without time delay. In all our patients who were scintigraphically examined after cranioplasty, we found no significant radionuclide accumulation in the contact sites between the prosthesis material and the skull bone, which speaks for a good tolerance of the plastic material used [81]. By contrast, by means of the "dynamic" scintigram, in patients who had brain mass displacement and hemisphere collapse before cranioplasty, an obviously delayed perfusion of the brain circulation on the still uncovered skull side has been observed (Fig. 17).

The strong concentration of activity of radionuclides, which is practically always visible in preoperative scintigrams of deeply pitted wounds, can be described as a "condensation effect". The brain tissue in the region of the bone gap is, as has already been discussed, compressed by the influence of atmospheric pressure [162]. Hence, the distribution of the radioactive substance is concentrated in a small space. As a consequence of this, an increased accumulation of activity in this area is observed.

This phenomenon can often serve as indication of the degree of brain compression in an uncovered skull [51]. An accumulation of radionuclides in the operating region still exists immediately after the performed cranioplasty and before the normalization of the intracranial situation. A calotte-shaped concentration of activity appears in the later postoperative course, because of the granulation tissue which develops around the acrylates. The lid is strongly

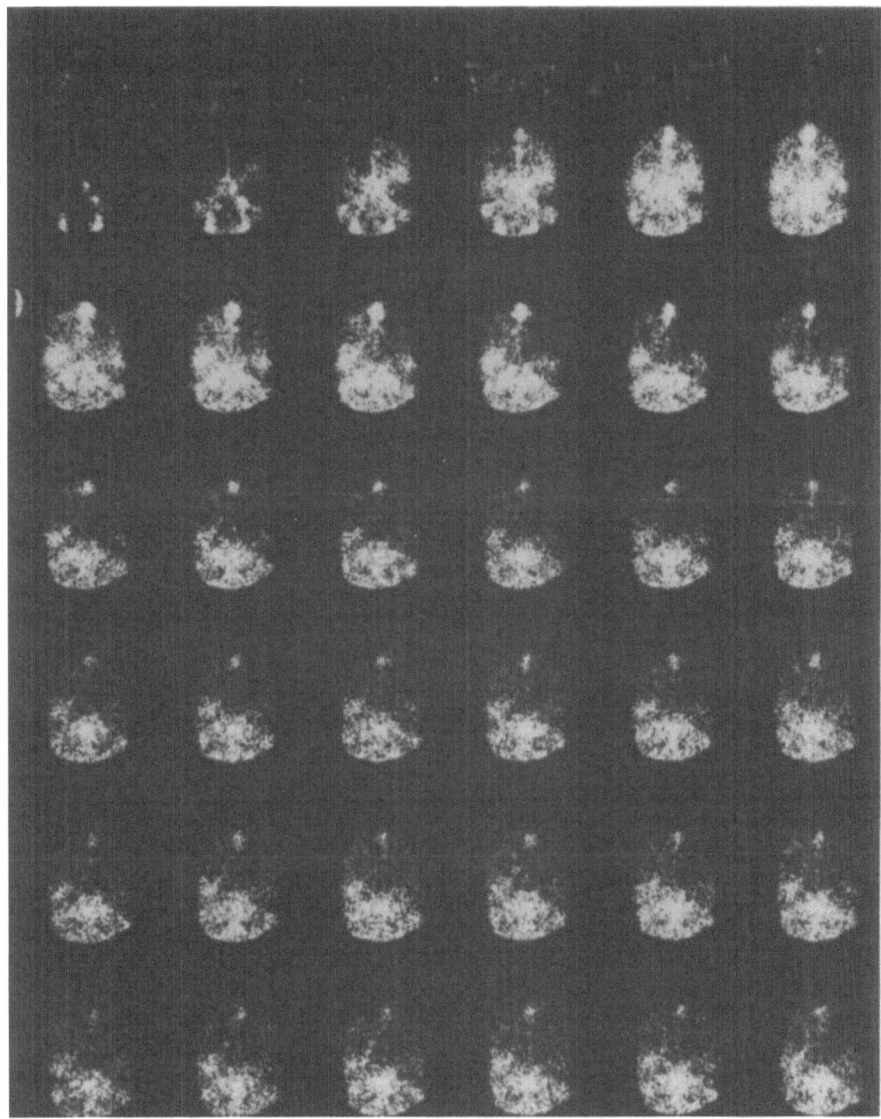

Fig. 17. A 55-year-old patient with a 6-month-old right temporo-parietal skull bone defect. Obvious delayed brain circulation on the right side. A radionuclide accumulation in the pitted skull defect region is visible in the last picture

vascularized; it shows an increased blood- and, therefore, also an increased activity flow.

Such findings, clearly indicating circulatory disturbances in the region of the uncovered and collapsed brain hemisphere, but showing a normal symmetrical perfusion pattern after cranioplasty, also confirm that cranioplasty

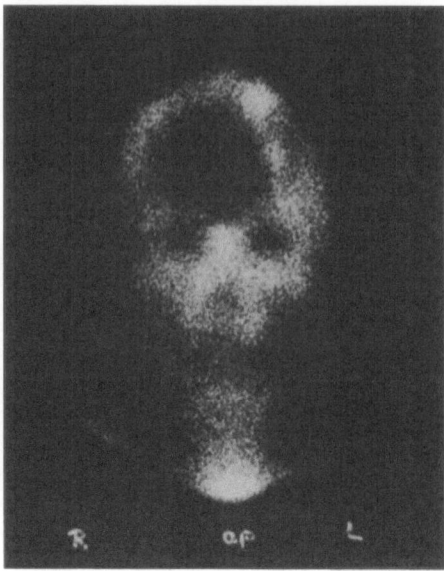

Fig. 18. Strong concentration of radionuclides in a skull defect of a 60-year-old patient after removal of an acute left parietal subdural haematoma

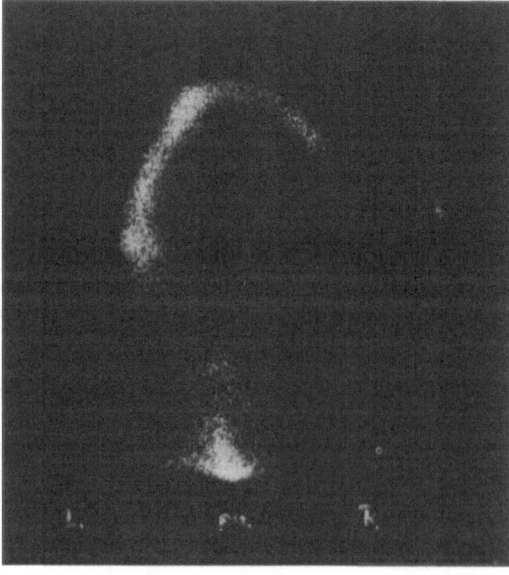

Fig. 19. The same patient as in Fig. 18, 3 months after cranioplasty

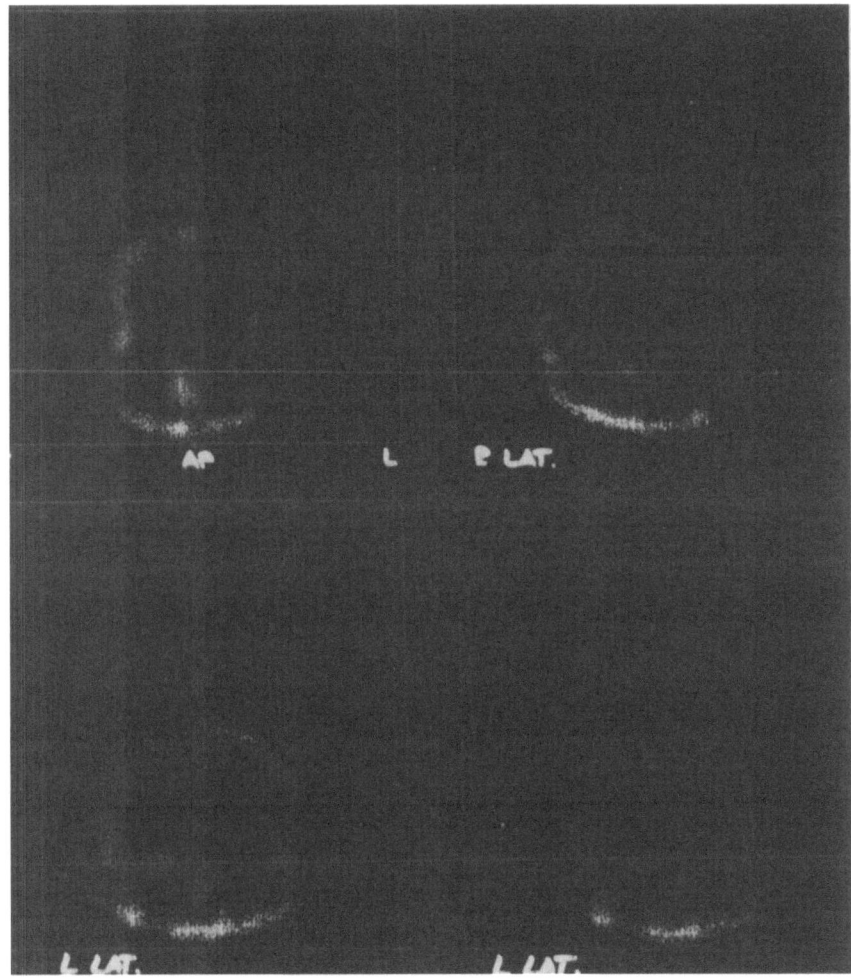

Fig. 20. The same patient as in Fig. 16. A slight calotte shaped radioactivity can be demonstrated 5 months after cranioplasty; the midline displacement does not exist anymore

exerts primary and foremost therapeutic effect, even though this is sometimes doubted [159, 161]. We noticed a normal symmetrical perfusion pattern in all our patients after cranioplasty.

Recently, it has been observed that a reduced brain circulation and thereby a deteriorated metabolic situation of the brain, leads to an extreme increase in cerebral lactate production. It is possible that such metabolic disturbances play a particular role in the development of psychoorganic syndrome which, sometimes, apart from neurological deficits, develops in large cranial defects [106].

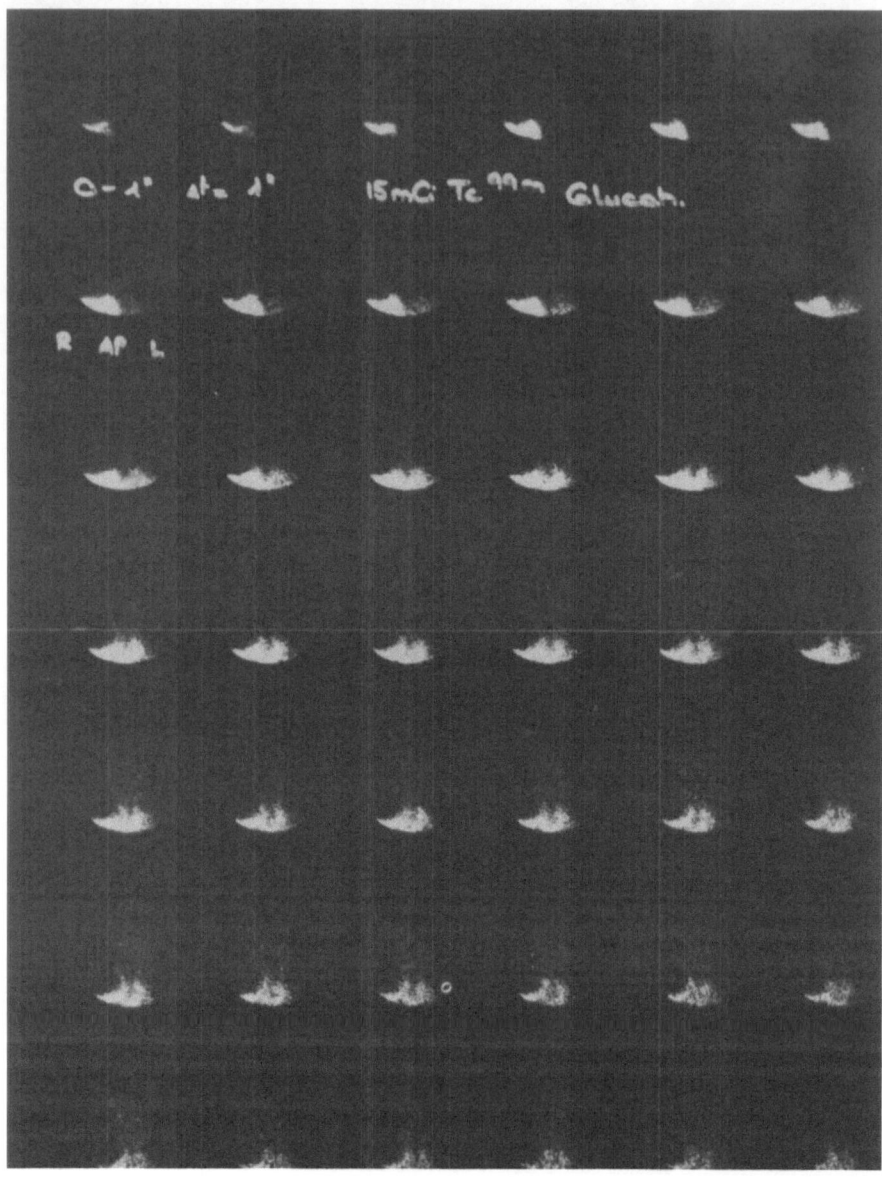

Fig. 21. The same patient as in Fig. 17, 5 months after cranioplasty. Symmetrical
perfusion pattern

V. Intracranial Pressure Changes Before and After Cranioplasty

The consequences of intracranial hypertension were already recognized in 1870 by Durett and by Cushing at the beginning of this century [7]. However, although of great importance, clinical recognition of intracranial hypertension is not often reliable [58]. For example, patients with slow growing brain tumours and a high intracranial pressure (ICP) may show only few clinical changes [7]. Recent introduction of continuous monitoring of intracranial pressure, which is independent of the subjective assessments of the physician, has not only enlarged the knowledge of pathogenesis, symptomatology and therapy of intracranial hypertension, but also partially allowed its correction.

According to current literature, intracranial pressure monitoring in patients with large cranial defects has so far not yet been the object of extensive clinical studies. This problem, however, takes an important place in reconstructive surgery.

Three methods of intracranial pressure monitoring have been developed: the *intraventricular,* the *subarachnoid* and the *epidural* method [50, 126, 130]. Currently, the first two methods, especially the most invasive intraventricular method, are loosing popularity. The introduction of the measuring probe into the lateral ventricle, in particular in the presence of fresh injuries and oedema, is not always easy and can cause additional serious damage to the brain tissue [75]. The not negligible infection rate and the formation of CSF fistulae caused by this method can often have severe consequences. Under these circumstances, also monitoring of ICP is more or less unreliable. Subarachnoid monitoring is not as invasive as the intraventricular method; nevertheless, long-term monitoring is not recommendable since, as with the intraventricular method, infections and fistulae can be provoked.

Epidural monitoring has more advantages and is, if properly used, not invasive. The dura remains intact so that the risk of meningitis and ventriculitis can be eliminated. The method is, therefore, suitable for continuous monitoring over a longer period. The uncertainty concerning the transposition of pressure through the dura might be regarded as a disadvantage. Recently, however, it has been shown that the epidural pressure measurements are equivalent to those of intraventricular and subdural methods, differing only by 3–5 mm Hg [75].

In our studies intracranial pressure was measured according to the principles as described by Gobiet [58–60]. The epidural pressure measuring device was composed of a hollow bolt (dome) and a transducer (Statham P 37 B) connected to electronic monitor (Hellige & Co., Germany) (Fig. 22). The device was implanted, mostly under local anaesthesia, into a burr-hole situated in the rear frontal region on the non-dominant side, 1–2 cm from the midline. A good haemostasis, especially of the dura, and a well fixed measuring instrument are the stipulations for unproblematic intracranial pressure monitoring. The control of zero-stability was performed twice daily.

It is to be mentioned that for the purpose of our study we found the Stratham transducer (Stratham Instr. Inc.) more suitable than the newly developed one of Gaeltec Ltd. Company (Scotland). Due to some technical advantages, the latter is today more currently used.

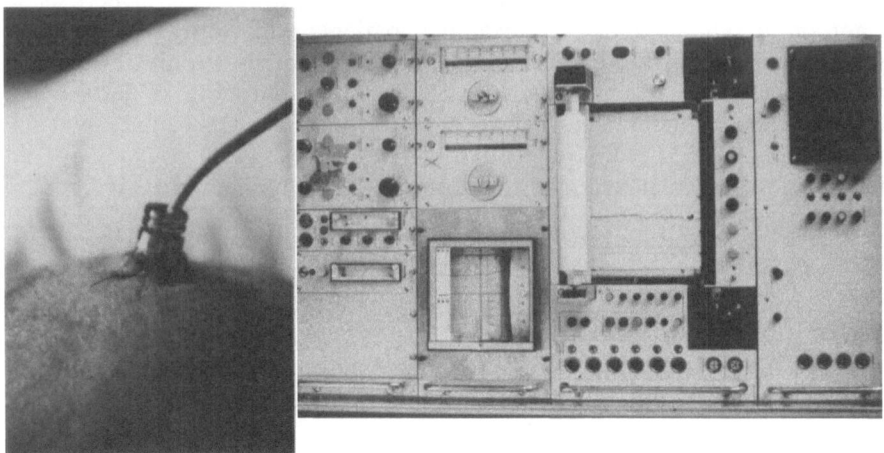

Fig. 22. A built-in pressure measuring device (Stratham) with electronic recorder

1. Casuistic

Of 103 patients with skull defects larger than $100 \, cm^2$, we used the epidural method of intracranial pressure monitoring before and after cranioplasty in 12 (11.7%) patients suitable for this method (no severe psychic changes, good general condition and good quality of the scalp). The average age of the examined patients was 37.8 years; the youngest was 19, the oldest 65 years old; 8 were males and 4 were females. In 3 patients the cranial defect was a consequence of a wound infection after a basal aneurysm operation, 2 patients had open craniocerebral injuries, and 7 patients an acute subdural haematoma with pronounced brain oedema. The intracranial pressure was monitored in minimum 1 and maximally 3 days before and 2–4 days after the surgery. The measurements were carried out in recumbent patients during the state of wakefulness as well as sleep. The pressure was graphically registered for 10–15 minutes per hour. The results of these investigations are summarized in Tables 6 and 7.

2. Preoperative Pressure Readings

According to the preoperative changes in intracranial pressure, 3 groups of patients could be distinguished (Tables 6, 7). The first group (4 patients)

Table 6. *Individual Values of Epidural Intracranial Pressure Before and After Cranioplasty*

Sex	Age	Diagnosis	Before cranioplasty			After cranioplasty		
			Average pressure in mm Hg recumbent		Average pressure values in 24 hrs.	Average pressure in mm Hg recumbent		Average pressure values in 24 hrs.
			Sleeping	Awake		Sleeping	Awake	
♂	52	Aneurysm of the anterior comm. artery	21	34	27.5	10	12	11
♂	32	Aneurysm of the anterior comm. artery and infection	18	30	24	5	10	7.5
♂	26	Acute subdural haematoma	10	24	17	5	9	7
♀	43	Acute subdural haematoma left parietal	12	18	15	3	7	5
♀	43	Acute subdural and intracerebral haematoma left parieto-occipital	10	18	14	6	10	8
♂	19	Acute subdural haematoma	12	15	13.5	6	10	8
♂	19	Acute subdural haematoma	10	15	12.5	5	10	7.5
♂	65	Acute subdural haematoma	9	8	8.5	7	5	6
♂	37	Open cranio-cerebral injury	6	10	8	0	6	3
♂	41	Open cranio-cerebral injury	5	10	7.5	6	8	7
♀	52	Aneurysm of the left middle cerebral artery	5	7	6	3	5	4
♀	25	Acute subdural haematoma	3	7	5	5	10	7.5

The values given in the table correspond to the average pressure measured after continuous recording during a minimum of 1 day and a maximum of 3 days (average value 1.8 days) before cranioplasty and 2 and 4 days, respectively, (average value 2.8 days) after cranioplasty. See text for methodological details.

Table 7. *Changes of the Epidural Intracranial Pressure Before and After Cranioplasty*

Number of patients	Mean age ($\bar{x}$)	Average values of intracranial pressure ($\bar{x} \pm SEM$) in mm Hg					
		Before cranioplasty			After cranioplasty		
		Recumbent			Recumbent		
		Sleeping	Awake	24 hour average	Sleeping	Awake	24 hour average
12	37.8 (19–65)	10.1 ±1.5	16.3 ±2.6	13.2 ±2.0	5.1 ±0.7	8.5 ±0.7	6.8 ±0.6

The statistical evaluation of the findings also shows that the postoperative intracranial pressure is significantly lower than the preoperative one (t = 3.70, df = 11, p < 0.005, Wilcoxon-test for paired comparison).

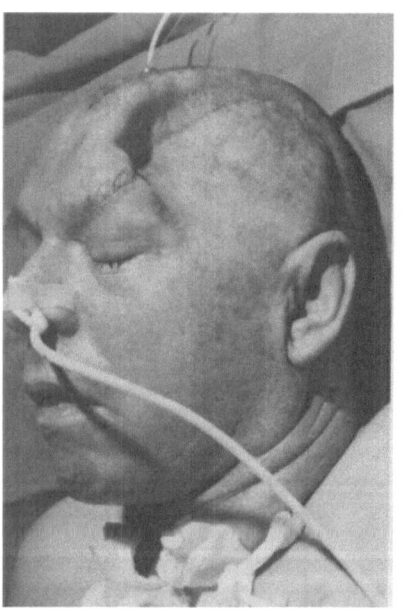

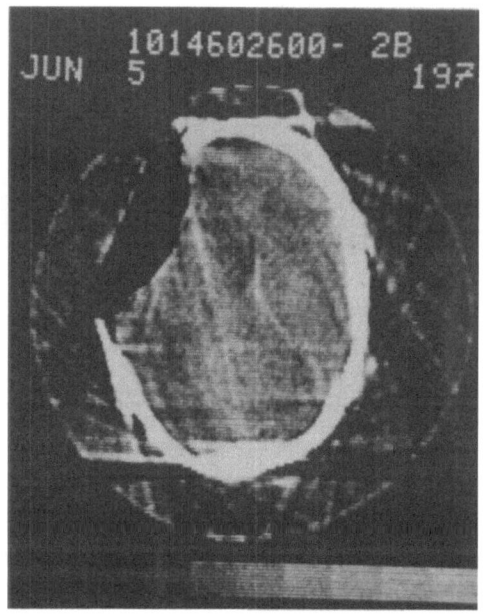

Fig. 23 a   Fig. 23 b

Fig. 23a. A 56-year-old patient 4 months after the clipping of an aneurysm of the anterior communicating artery. The cranial bone was removed 1 week postoperatively because of the wound infection. Marked pitting of the wound with a right hemiplegia, aphasia and somnolence

Fig. 23b. CT: obvious brain mass displacement towards the right. The intracranial pressure was 27 mm Hg (36.7 cm H_2O) in this phase

showed pressure readings between 20.4 (minimum) and 36.7 mm Hg (maximum) (19.5 and 32 cm H_2O respectively).

All these patients had large cranial defects with extensively pitted sunken-in skin flaps (Figs. 23a, b; 24a, b). Moreover, all of them showed severe neurological deficits. Two patients were in the state of somnolence.

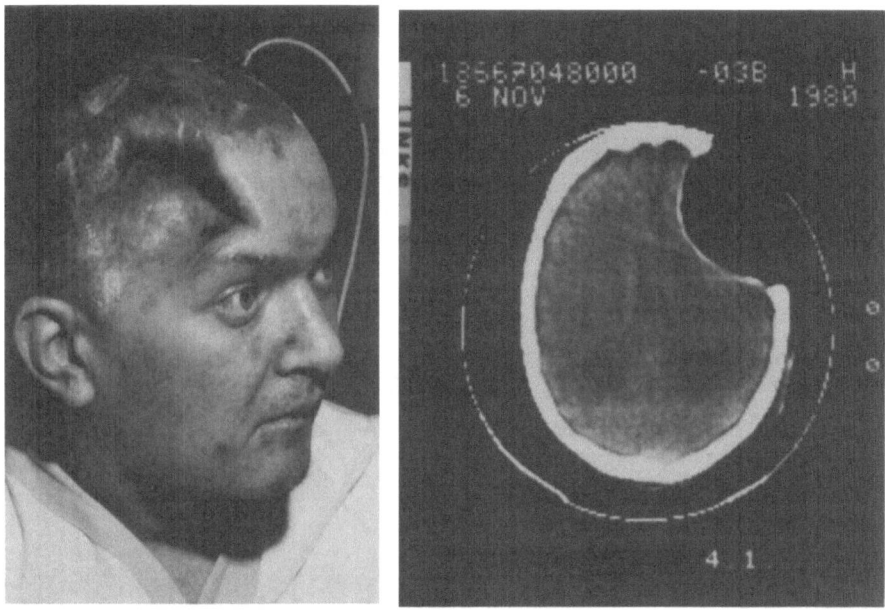

Fig. 24a   Fig. 24b

Fig. 24a. A 32-year-old patient 9 months after clipping the anterior communicating
         artery. The skull bone was removed because of the wound infection

Fig. 24b. Brain mass displacement towards the left and a POS developed some
2 months postoperatively. The intracranial pressure read 24 mm Hg (32.6 cm H_2O)

In the second group of patients (n = 3) the intracranial pressures were at the upper limit of normality: 10 and 15 mm Hg (13 and 19.5 cm H_2O). These patients were characterized by smaller brain mass displacements and less pitting of the skin flaps. In general, the neurological changes were also less dramatic than in the first group. Nevertheless, one patient showed serious psychoorganic syndrome (POS) with aphasia and hemiparesis. One patient had hemiparesis of a moderate degree and another one showed no neurological changes at all. The illustrative example of a patient from this group is presented in Figs. 25a, b.

In a third group of 5 patients, intracranial pressure was in average below 10 mm Hg (13 cm H_2O). The patients of this group, with practically normal

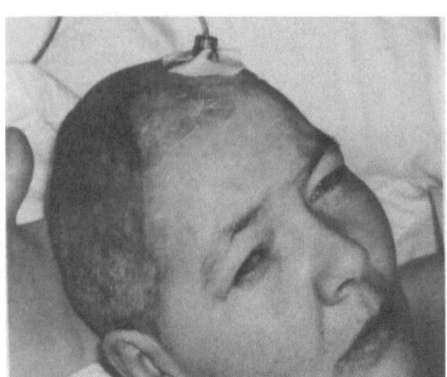
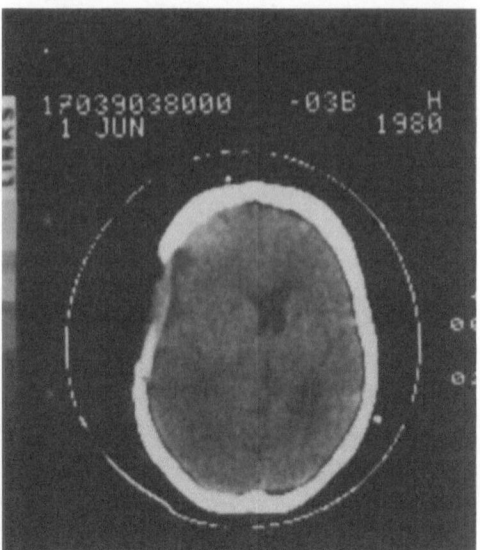

Fig. 25a   Fig. 25b

Fig. 25a. A 42-year-old patient 4 months after the removal of an acute subdural haematoma

Fig. 25b. CT: brain mass displacement and hemisphere deformation. The clinical picture is dominated by aphasia, psychoorganic syndrome and hemisyndrome

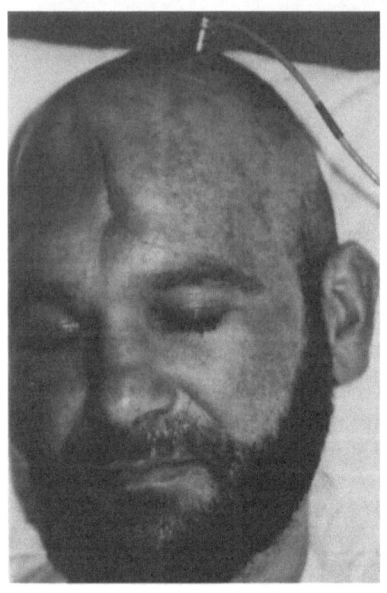

Fig. 26a   Fig. 26b

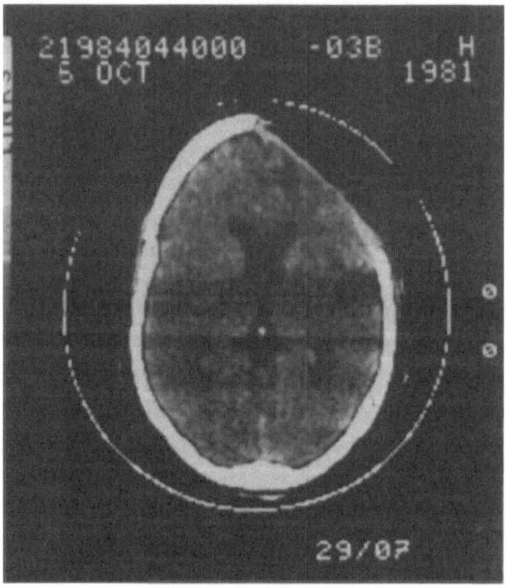

Fig. 26a. A 37-year-old patient 9 months after open craniocerebral injury, neurologically and psychologically without pathological findings

Fig. 26b. CT: slight hemisphere deformation without brain mass displacement or any other changes

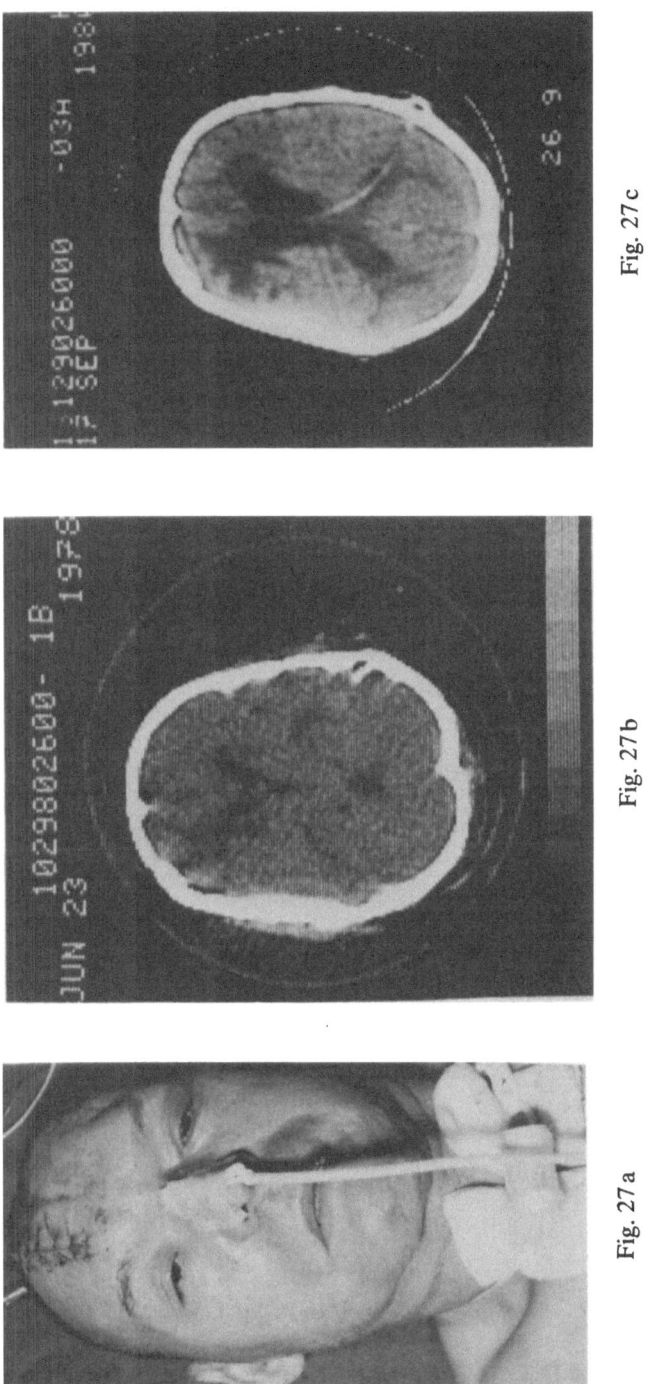

Fig. 27 c

Fig. 27 b

Fig. 27 a

Fig. 27a. The same patient as in Fig. 23a, 3 weeks after cranioplasty

Fig. 27b. CT: brain mass displacement is almost compensated, brain hemisphere is expanded, the intracranial pressure sank from preoperatively 27.5 mm Hg to 11 mm Hg

Fig. 27c. CT: an AV shunt (Pudenz) operation was performed 2 years after the cranioplasty because of hydrocephalus internus

preoperative intracranial pressures, were predominantly without neurological changes and showed only a slight pitting of the skin flap without brain mass displacement and only minimal brain compression (Figs. 26 a, b). We detected a slight POS in only one patient of this group.

3. Postoperative Pressure Readings

The preoperatively implanted pressure measuring device was not removed during the surgery, and the monitoring was continued postoperatively in the same manner. The pressure normalized itself after the cranioplasty in all patients of the first group, who had an elevated intracranial pressure. In one case a preoperative pressure of 27.5 mm Hg sank to 11 mm Hg (14 cm H$_2$O) postoperatively (Figs. 27 a, b, c).

The normalization of intracranial pressure in these patients was paralleled by marked clinical improvement. Hemiplegia in one patient showed clear-cut signs of recovery, and the pre-existing psychoorganic syndrome regressed in all patients. In the patients of the second group, with average pressure readings between 10 and 15 mm Hg, postoperative pressure control showed a clear-cut tendency towards normalization. In one of these patients mean pressure higher than 10 mm Hg was recorded. However, severe neurological changes observed in one of these patients before the surgery (see above and Fig. 25) failed to improve (Figs. 28 a, b).

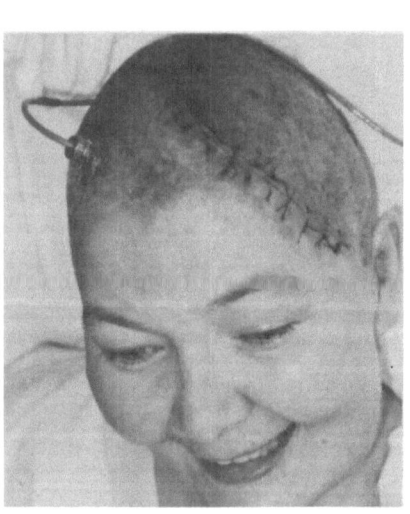 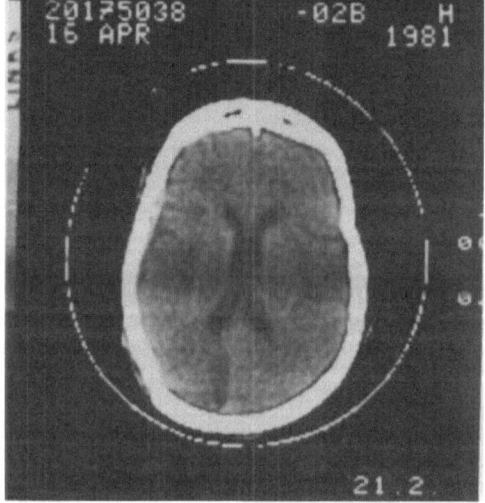

Fig. 28 a   Fig. 28 b

Fig. 28 a, b. The same patient as in Fig. 25 a one week after cranioplasty. The intracranial condition has practically normalized (see Fig. 28 b CT); nevertheless the neurological findings (aphasia, POS, hemiparesis) showed no improvement at this time

4. *Pathophysiology of Increased Intracranial Pressure in Uncovered Skull Defects*

The mechanisms of the formation of the deeply pitted skin flap, which causes considerable difficulties, is not yet completely understood. According to the law of Monroe – Kelly there exists a constant proportion between the constituents (blood, CSF and brain) of the inner cranium [31, 134]. When these elements remain in normal proportions to each other, no large intracranial changes can take place. Moreover, a loss or change of one of the

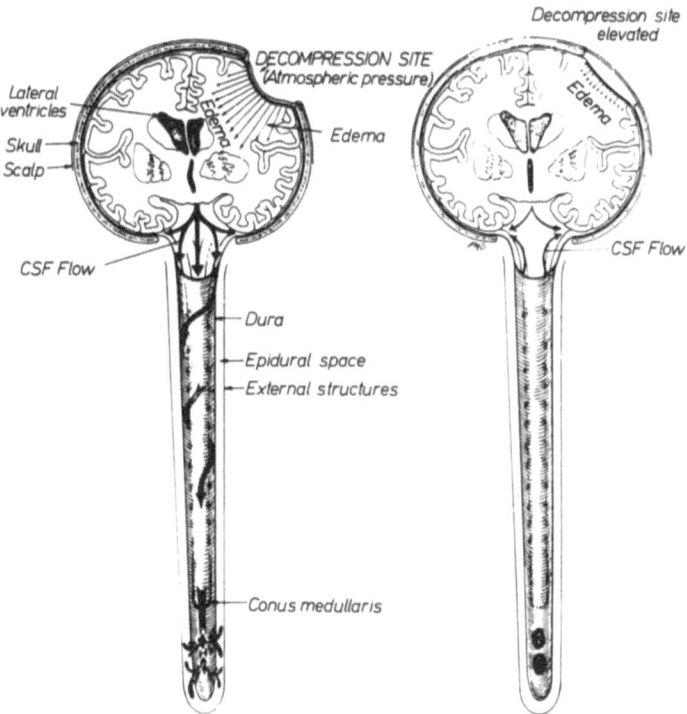

Fig. 29. Schematic presentation of the effect of atmospheric pressure upon uncovered cranial defect (modification of the original presentation by Guido [68])

constituents is compensated by either the same or by enlargement of another element of the cranial contents [124]. Since the brain mass can be displaced to only a limited extent, an increase or decrease in the intracranial contents is achieved by changes in the volume of CSF and, in addition, by changes in the filled volume of the blood vessels [51].

After a decompressive trepanation with bone flap removal, the normal conditions within the brain cavity are impaired. The inner cranium is no more separated and insulated from the outer influences: the only barriers separating the brain from the external environment are now the dura and the skin. The atmospheric pressure can act directly on an almost unprotected brain (Fig. 29).

It is generally assumed that the pitted and retracted skin flaps are the consequence of the resulting differences in the outer and inner pressures [68, 162, 186, 187]. Moreover, it is suggested that the brain mass displacement and collapsing of the ventricles develop because of the constant influence of the external atmospheric pressure upon the unprotected brain. The CSF as the most mobile component of the brain constituents, which is able to pass freely in and out of the brain cavity through foramen occipitale magnum, is squeezed out of the ventricle system. Its volume within the cavity, therefore, decreases.

It must be stressed, however, that the mechanisms by which these intracranial changes are generated, were until recently largely unknown [159]. In the past, the invasive investigation methods only available at that time, like carotis angiography and air-encephalography, were not easy to use and, therefore, seldom practised. Moreover, the deleterious effects as well as the severity of the syndrome developing in large skull defects with pitted skin flap

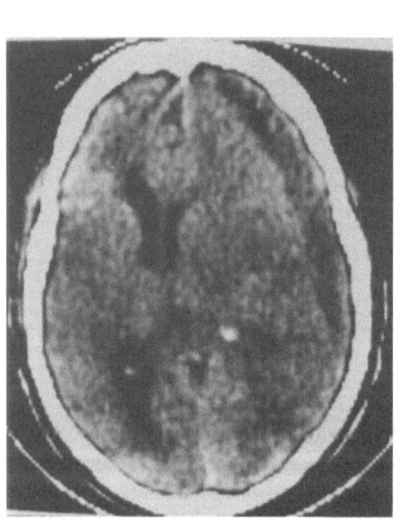
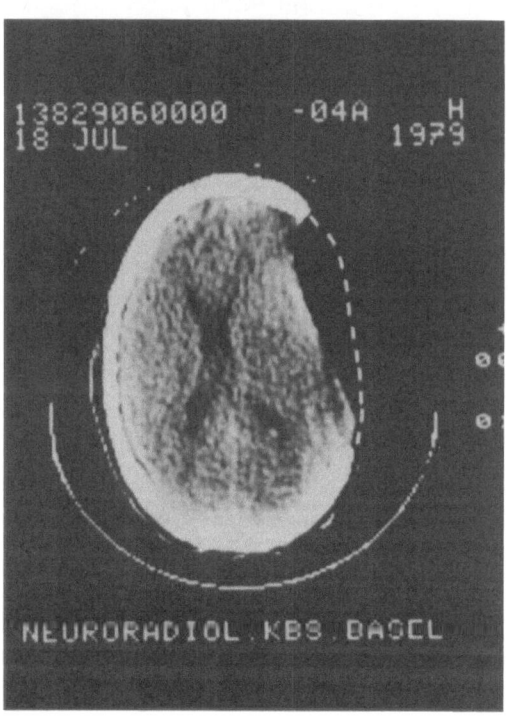

Fig. 30a   Fig. 30b

Fig. 30a. Hemisphere compression, brain mass displacement with ventricle deformation: usual picture of raised intracranial pressure in space occupying processes (here: chronic subdural haematoma)

Fig. 30b. Cranial bone defect in a 19-year-old patient, 4 months after removal of an acute subdural haematoma. The same intracranial situation as in Fig. 30a but here without the intracranial space occupying process. (The same pathoanatomic changes develop in both cases) were generally underestimated. The development and introduction of computer tomography as a non-invasive and fast method has for the first time permitted more accurate assessment of intracranial changes. Severe hemisphere deformations with brain mass displacements and ventricle collapse were visualized. Only then did it become obvious that the intracranial state plays an important role also in the origin of neurological and psychic symptoms accompanying such defects and handicapping the patients in their everyday life. Some unexpected facts were also revealed.

We remind that, initially, a reduction of the raised intracranial pressure was achieved by means of a pressure relieving trepanation (decompressive craniotomy). In the course of the time a particular clinical picture develops: the skin flap over the skull defect slowly retracts, the proportions within the cranium change and, eventually, a new state characterized by brain mass displacement, brain compression and ventricle deformation develops. No doubt, this picture appears very much similar to the conditions observed in raised intracranial pressure due to space occupying processes. In this respect is illustrative Fig. 30 (a, b). By comparing the left and the right figures, no substantial difference between the skull CTs of the two examples can be found. Both patients showed signs of increased intracranial pressure, and the clinical picture was similar in that they displayed left hemiparesis. The similarity of clinical and neurological as well as CT findings strongly suggested that at least in some patients an increase, and not decrease, in intracranial pressure develops after a certain period of time. Continuous monitoring of the intracranial pressure, which was performed in our patients, substantiated this assumption. Cranial repair led to the stabilization of intracranial pressure as well as its normalization in 75% of the examined patients (Fig. 31). In all probability neurological and psychic symptoms found preoperatively in these cases could be also attributed to such increased pressure.

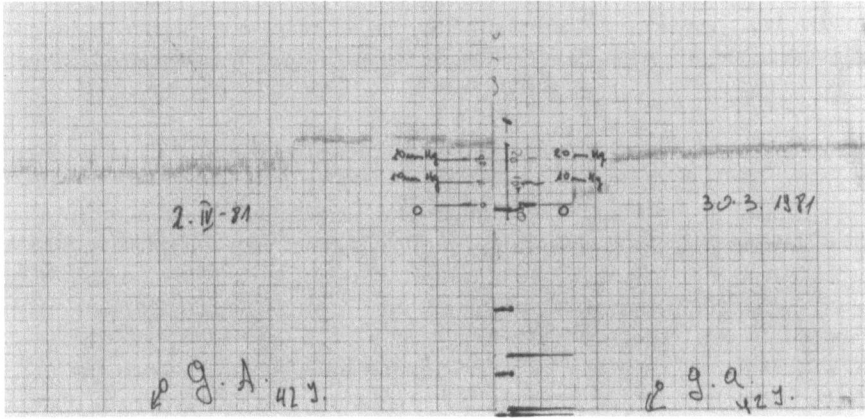

Fig. 31. Intracranial pressure decreased to 10 mm Hg after cranioplasty (picture left). Intracranial pressure of 20 mm Hg before the operation, rhythmically current β-waves (picture right)

4*

As stressed before, several authors hypothesized that the origin of the sinking skin-flap and consecutive disturbances could be explained by the difference in the atmospheric and intracranial pressure. This explanation, however, does not seem entirely plausible. It is a known fact that the difference between the in- and outside pressures is rather small. It should be, however, large if it is to be considered as responsible for the extensive intracranial changes observed in uncovered skull defects. In our opinion, a "scar

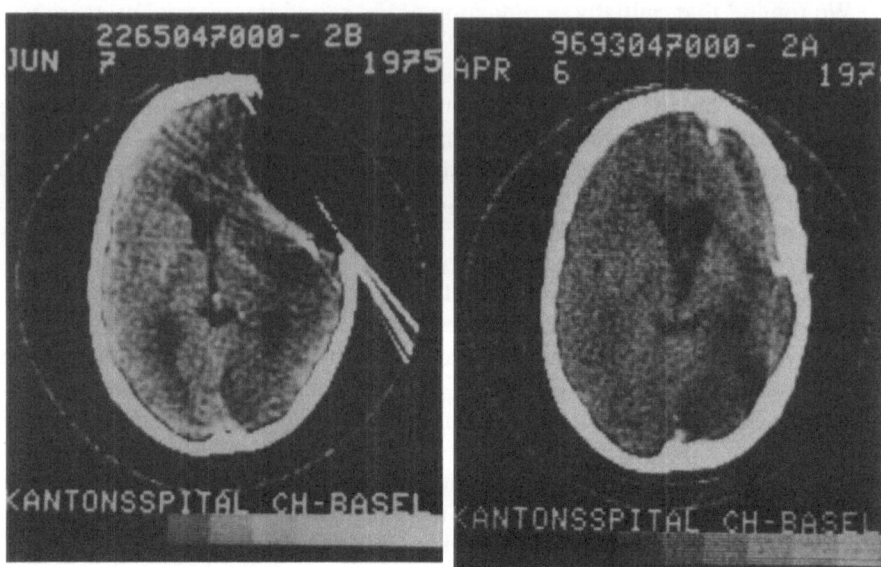

Fig. 32 a   Fig. 32 b

Fig. 32a. A 28-year-old patient after removal of an acute subdural haematoma. Marked brain mass displacement with ventricle deformation and pitting of the brain

Fig. 32b. The expansion of the brain and the normalization of the brain mass displacement after intralumbar injection of Ringer's solution (condition 10 months later)

plate" which is formed between the brain cortex, dura and skin plays also a role in the development of the syndrome. In the course of the time it retracts and protrudes inwards and thus reduces the intracranial space. Moreover, as shown by our systematic scintigraphy studies (see before), the filled volume of the blood vessels is changed and the brain circulation clearly retarded. In an already reduced intracranial space, brain mass displacement and brain compression may, therefore, develop.

Certainly, the complex mechanisms of the intracranial pressure and other changes are, even so, not satisfactorily explained and remain to be further explored. The importance of the differences in the intracranial and atmospheric pressure also cannot be neglected.

In the majority of cases, as already stressed, cranioplasty, which eliminates the influence of external factors, restores the physiological conditions in the

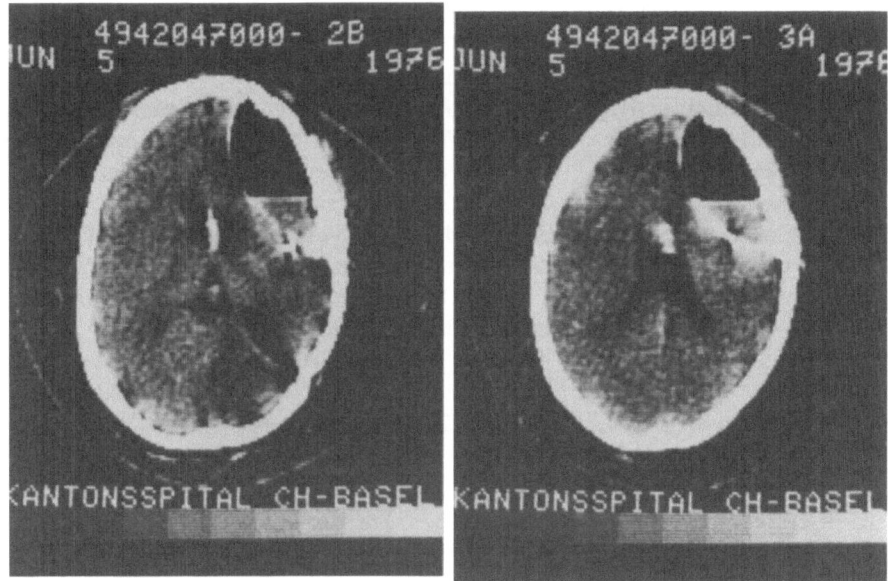

Fig. 33a   Fig. 33b

Fig. 33a, b. An infected haematoma in the epidural space with an unexpanded brain after cranioplasty. In spite of intraoperative expansion and normalization the brain retracted itself again a short time after the cranioplasty and formed a hollow space under the plastic. Atrioventricular CSF shunt is visible on the right

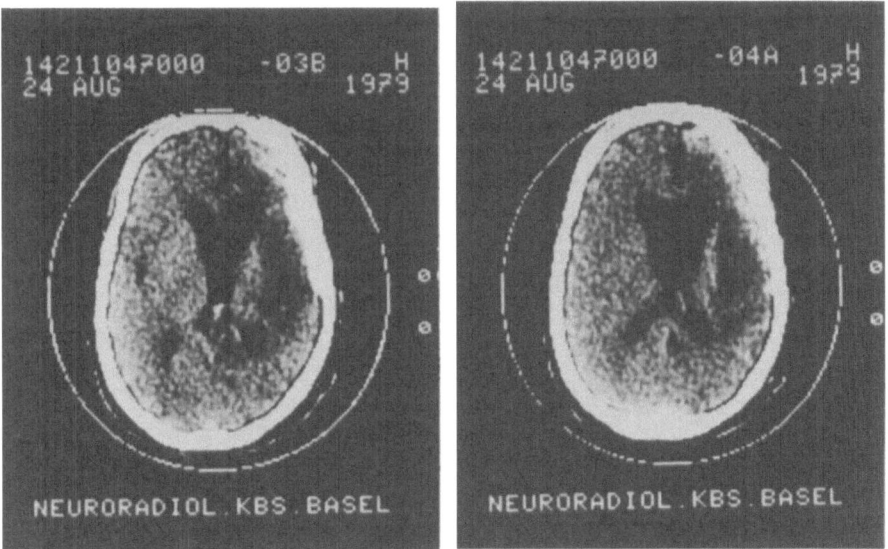

Fig. 34a   Fig. 34b

Fig. 34a, b. CT of the skull: the same patient as in Fig. 32, 4 years later. No changes, ventricle configuration with a slight hydrocephalus

brain cavity [112, 124]. However, in some cases an immediate expansion of the brain is not achieved, possibly because of the relative "loss" of the CSF. This loss could be compensated by an appropriate amount of warm (35–37 °C) physiological saline or Ringer's solution infused via a catheter inserted into the lumbar space before the operation (Figs. 32a, b). Sometimes, however, this treatment, even if repeated, could also prove to be unsuccessful (Figs. 33a, b). Under these conditions, the cranioplasty is encountering considerably more intra- as well as postoperative problems. Nevertheless, the possibility of infection caused by the retention of the serum or blood in the hollow space is hereby considerably reduced. If all the same an infection with epidural empyema develops, revision and removal of cranioplasty is indicated.

Although some authors believe that replacement of CSF has only temporary effects [116, 168], in our experience this intervention was of long-lasting benefit (Figs. 34a, b). The exceptions are patients where, because of the development of hydrocephalus, a CSF shunt had to be performed. In such cases proper expansion of the brain could not be obtained even after repeated injections of Ringer's solution into the subdural space. The desired correction was achieved only after tying or removal of the shunt.

C. Surgical Procedures and Techniques of Cranial Repair

I. Indications for Cranioplasty

As early as 1943 Seiffert pointed out to the lack of informations in the published literature clearly stating the indications and reasons for repairing cranial defects. The same author principally refused cranioplasty as a surgical treatment procedure, "except for a few almost negligible exceptions". This attitude of a then well-known author illustrates how little importance was attached to cranioplasty in the past. Even more, in 1931, in his monograph on the fate of gunshot-wounded patients, Vogler, expressing his concern about cranial defect repair, warned of cranioplasty. He argued that 15–16% of the operated non-epileptics develop epileptic fits after the surgery. Krüger [105] suggested that the main reason for the plastic repair of skull defects was to eliminate the deformation, especially in the fronto-basal region (see [10]). As a matter of fact, not long ago, cranioplasty in the area of the convexity was carried out rather rarely and primarily because of the "favourable influence on epilepsy" [3, 43, 53].

Many authors also emphasized the cosmetic point of view, mechanical factors and subjective discomfort as indications for the repair of the skull defects [142, 169].

Based on our experience, the indications for cranioplasty can be divided into four groups [159]:

1. prevention or elimination of hemisphere collapses or midline displacements (curative effect),
2. treatment of space occupying CSF cysts,
3. protection against mechanical influences,
4. cosmetic restoration.

The time to perform cranioplasty is largely determined by the nature as well as the origin of the defect. Congenital and neoplastic cranial defects can mostly be primarily covered. Conversly, traumatic skull defects should not be repaired unless at least 3–6 months after the healing of the primary wound have passed. It is advisable to wait even longer (over 12 months) if there are signs of the rarefaction of the bone caused by secondary infections producing osteomyelitis [73, 74, 79, 142].

Prevention or elimination of hemisphere collapses or midline displacement as well as treatment of space occupying CSF cysts are two new important indications which deserve to be added to the classical indications for cranioplasty.

1. Prevention of Hemisphere Collapse

The fact that cranioplasty could serve as a preventive measure or correction of hemisphere deformation and ventricle collapse, developing in large skull defects and frequently causing neurological impairments, has been recently indicated by some authors [162]. As stressed before, the latter are primarily

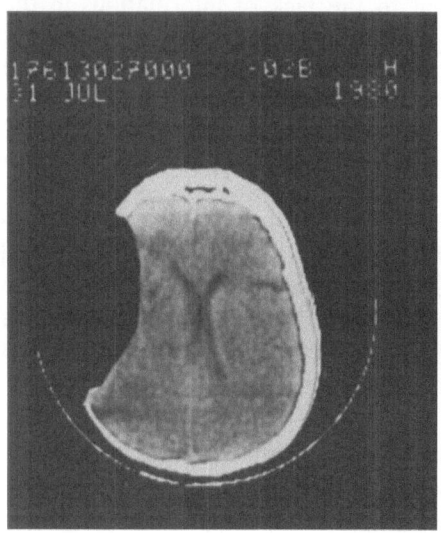 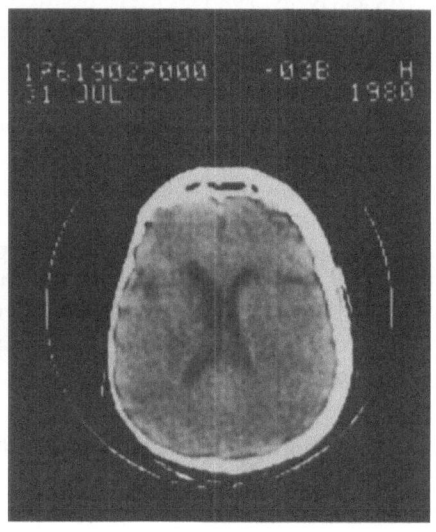

Fig. 35 a   Fig. 35 b

Fig. 35 a. A 53-year-old patient showing hemisphere compression with brain mass displacement 2 months after removal of an acute subdural haematoma

Fig. 35 b. Expansion of the brain and reversal of the brain mass displacement the *very same day of the cranioplasty*

observed in patients in which large craniotomies because of acute traumatic hemorrhagies or tumourous infiltrations into the bone have been performed. The disabling symptoms mostly persist over several months.

Thoroughful studies and analysis of this problem by means of computer tomography have shown that cranioplasty exerts a beneficial normalizing effect on intracranial changes in such cases. Even when a CT control is not possible in the early postoperative stage because of organizational or other reasons, several observations indicate that the correction of the lateral displacement may occur within a few days or, sometimes, immediately after cranioplasty [159] (Figs. 35a, b). Parallel to the correction of brain mass displacement, the neurological symptoms usually also show a tendency to normalize. Several examples have confirmed that the reversal of the hemisphere collapse and brain mass displacement, as seen in the computer tomogram, is accompanied by a positive postoperative clinical progress [159, 162] (Figs. 36a, b).

In the following the curative effect of cranioplasty is illustrated by several examples.

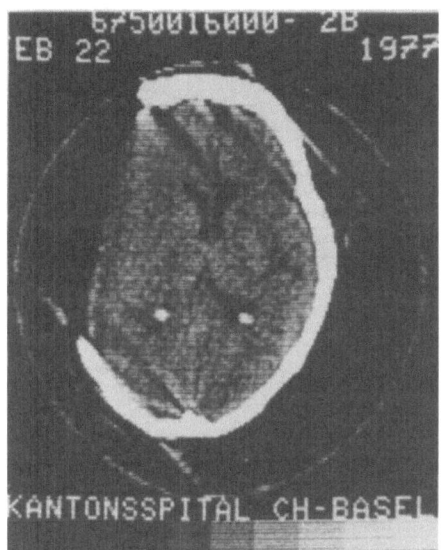 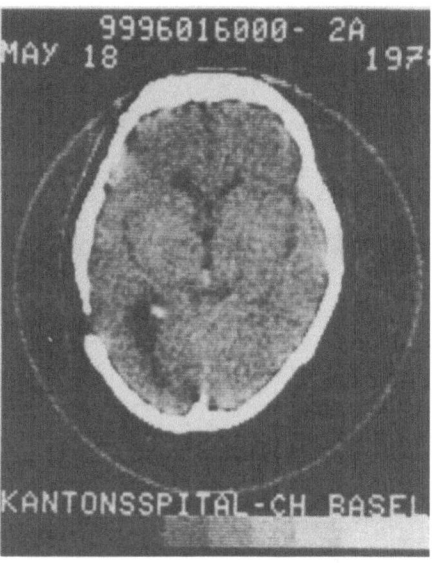

Fig. 36a   Fig. 36b

Fig. 36a. 61-year-old patient with a large skull defect after removal of an acute subdural haematoma. Marked brain mass displacement towards the left with hemisphere compression. A right-sided hemisyndrome appeared 4 months after the removal of the haematoma

Fig. 36b. Cranioplasty 14 months later with the patient's own bone. Brain mass displacement and brain compression regressed. The hemisyndrome regressed within a week

1.1 Case Reports

Case No 1:

A 51-year-old patient suffered from chronic subdural haematoma complicated by intraoperative bleeding. The cranial repair surgery with acrylates had been performed in another hospital 2 years before admission to our clinic; later on, the prosthesis had, however, to be removed because of

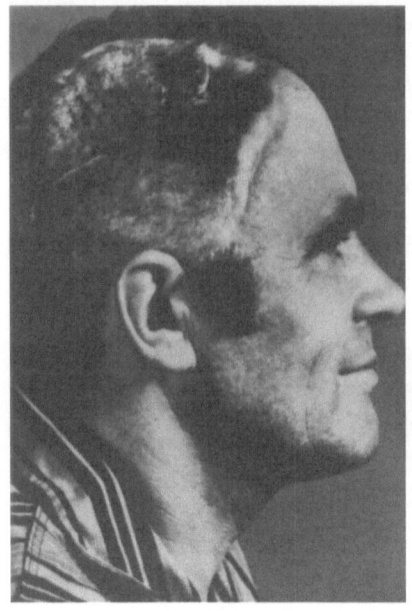

Fig. 37 a

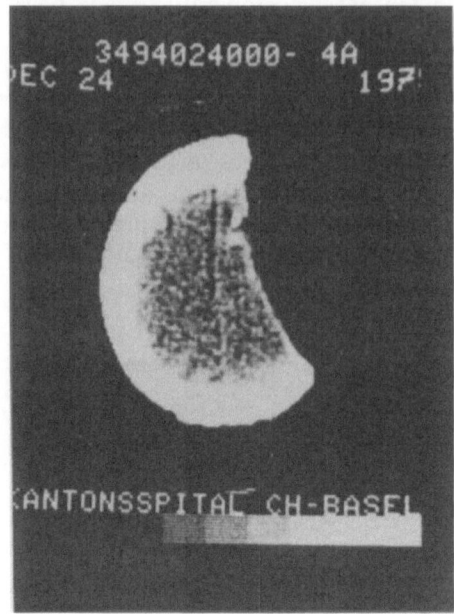

Fig. 37 b

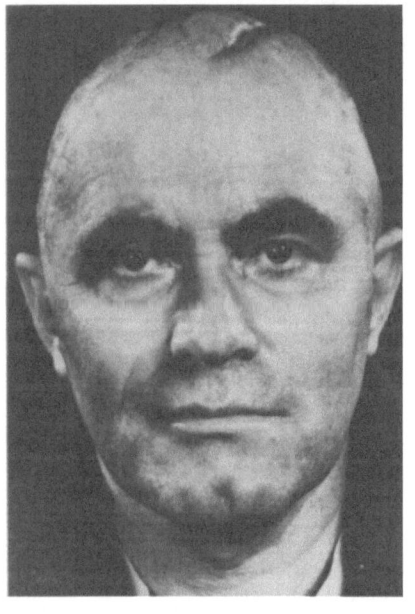

Fig. 38 a

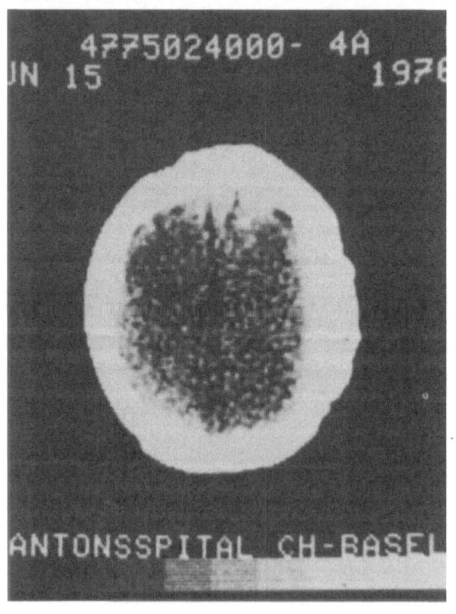

Fig. 38 b

infection. During the last months a marked brain collapse was accompanied by a considerable, progressive hemiparesis on the opposite side of the defect and by severe psychoorganic syndrome. All the symptoms almost completely regressed after the renewed repair of the defect. However, again the plastic had to be removed because of a wound infection, and the hemisphere collapse and the hemiplegia promptly reappeared. Following definitive, successful surgical treatment, the neurological status normalized again (Figs. 37a, b; 38a, b).

Case No 2:

In November 1976, a 64-year-old lady was involved in a car accident. She was admitted to the hospital because of brain contusion with an acute subdural haematoma, left temporo-parietal and a right-sided fracture of the base of the

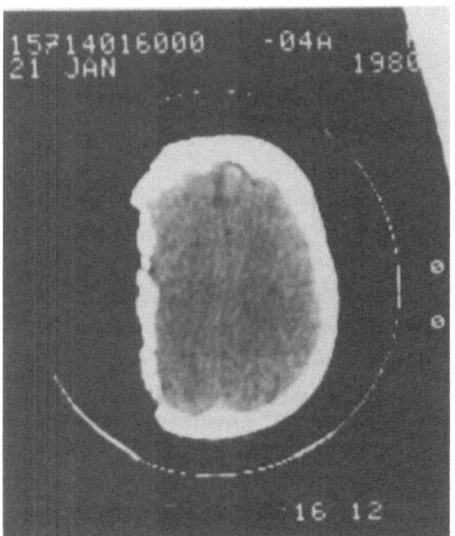 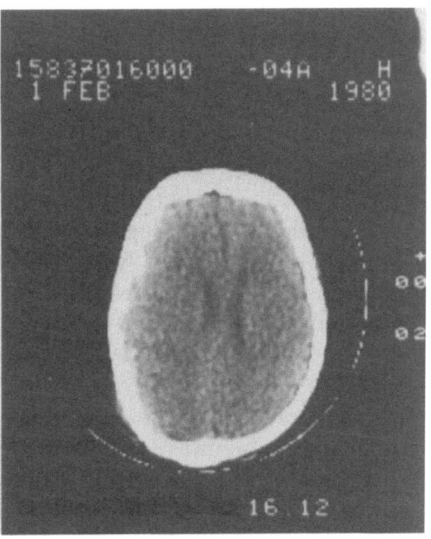

Fig. 39a   Fig. 39b

Fig. 39a. The patient's own bone implanted 3 years before, markedly hollowed and absorbed to a large extent, visible compression on the left hemisphere

Fig. 39b. After cranioplasty with acrylate (Palacos® R with Gentamycin). Normalization of the intracranial situation

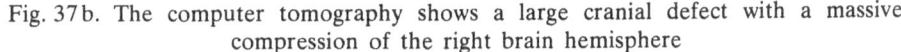

Fig. 37a. A 51-year-old patient after several operations for a chronic subdural haematoma with following wound infection. 4 months after the operation a POS and a left-sided hemisyndrome developed

Fig. 37b. The computer tomography shows a large cranial defect with a massive compression of the right brain hemisphere

Fig. 38a, b. The same patient as in Fig. 37a three weeks after cranioplasty with Palacos® R: the hemiparesis had completely regressed, the POS symptoms showed a tendency of disappearing as well. The computer tomography of the skull shows a complete expansion of the brain skull. After craniotomy the haematoma was removed. Postoperatively, slight right-sided hemiparesis and slight speech difficulties remained. About 3 months later the skull defect was repaired by means of the patient's own bone. The patient fully recovered thereafter. In 1978, probably coinciding with the absorption of the patient's own bone, progressive gait disturbances developed. The patient complained during this period more and more frequently about disequilibrium; increasing signs of paraparesis of the lower extremities developed. In 1980 she was again admitted to the hospital. At admission the patient showed severe gait disturbances. Cognitive deficits with a superimposed depression were also evident. Cranioplasty with acrylate was performed. At surgery, large depressed piece of bone disintegrated by absorption and causing brain compression was found on the left side. The palacos prosthesis was implanted without complications. During the postoperative course her clinical condition improved rapidly. An impressive regression of the severe ataxia as well as an improvement of her mental state was observed (Figs. 39a, b).

Case No 3:

A 52-year-old patient with an aneurysm of the left a. communicans posterior developed progressive clouding of consciousness a week after the clipping of the aneurysm. A subdural haematoma which appeared postoperatively was removed and a bone flap decompression was undertaken because of brain oedema. In the further postoperative progress, a deeply pitted bone gap and rapidly developing midbrain symptoms with coma, staring pupils and extension spasms were observed. After changing the body position of the patient (head lower than the body) these symptoms, however, disappeared within a few minutes. At the same time, the large pitting of the skin flap regressed too. In the sitting position or with the raised head, besides the sunken-in skin flap and the brain collapse, a CSF loss was evident. Both these components gave a clinical picture of severe strangulation. After the surgical repair of the defect, the patient recovered rapidly.

Case No 4:

In a 31-year-old patient total absorption of the patient's own bone took place within 18 months after cranioplasty, consecutive to the removal of an acute subdural haematoma. A pronounced left hemiparesis and psychic changes developed in the patient who, until then, had shown no neurological changes. Marked skin flap pitting with hemisphere collapse and brain mass displacement was revealed by means of the CT. After the renewed repair of the skull defect – this time with acrylate – the left sided paresis as well as the psychoorganic symptoms showed obvious tendency to regress. Upon discharge from the hospital, the patient was almost symptom free.

2. Treatment of CSF Cysts

The second important indication for cranioplasty, which can be diagnosed and followed by computer tomography, is the treatment of the space occupying CSF cysts. CSF cysts are occasionally seen in the following cases: after decompression craniotomy because of acute subdural haematoma or after intracerebral bleeding communicating with the subdural space. Furthermore,

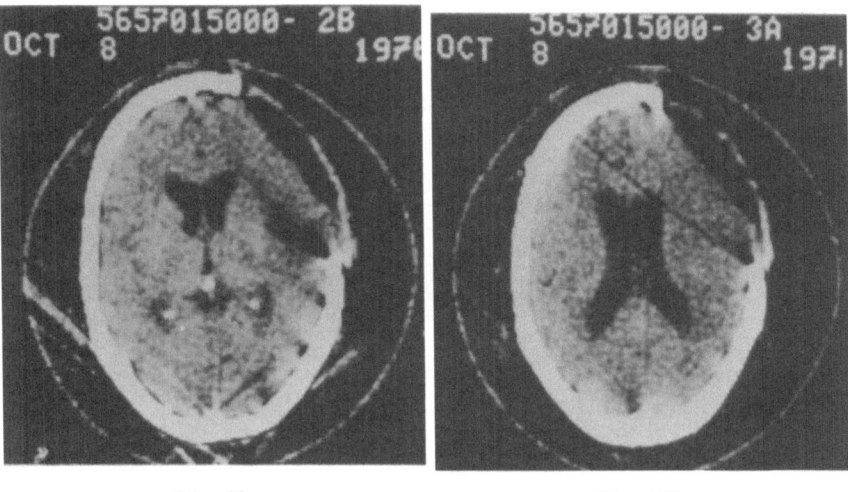

Fig. 40a   Fig. 40b

Fig. 40a, b. CSF cyst in the right frontal region and bone flap decompression after the removal of an acute subdural haematoma

they develop after bone flap decompression because of brain oedema and, last but not least, after decompressions because of the enlargement of dura due to severe contusions of the brain, malignant brain oedema and marked brain mass displacement. These cysts develop in the postoperative period and are sometimes space occupying [159] (Figs. 40 and 41a, b). The formation of the CSF cysts could be pathophysiologically explained by a disturbance in the CSF circulation. It is known that after every subarachnoid bleeding, of either spontaneous or traumatic origin, an aseptic leptomeningeal reaction with adhesions occurs. The latter is a consequence – as it is nearly always happening in the cerebral contusions – of the extravasation of blood into the CSF and chemical irritation of the pia mater. Adhesions in the region of the basal cisterne produce disturbances in the CSF passage and absorption [47, 68]. As soon as CSF production exceeds CSF absorption, every free space in the intracranium is replenished by the increasing volume of the CSF. The removal of the cyst and the consecutive cranioplasty favour the regression of the brain mass displacement and the expansion of the brain; the intracranial state returns to normal.

Occasionally, due to the above mentioned reasons, hydrocephalus internus could also develop. This postcontusional "hydrocephalus male resorptivus" has not been well known until recently. It is still diagnosed too rarely [104]. But, in general such hydrocephalus is more and more frequent, since the current intensive postoperative therapy prevents the fatal outcome of patients with severe brain injuries, which was years ago still unavoidable. In the treatment of postcontusional hydrocephalus it is essential to restore the balance in the CSF dynamics. For this purpose an atrio-ventriculo-peritoneal CSF shunt must be introduced.

The frequency of postcontusional hydrocephalus in our population of patients with craniocerebral injuries (n = 116) was about 15% (n = 17). In all of them we have performed CSF drainage in addition to cranial repair surgery.

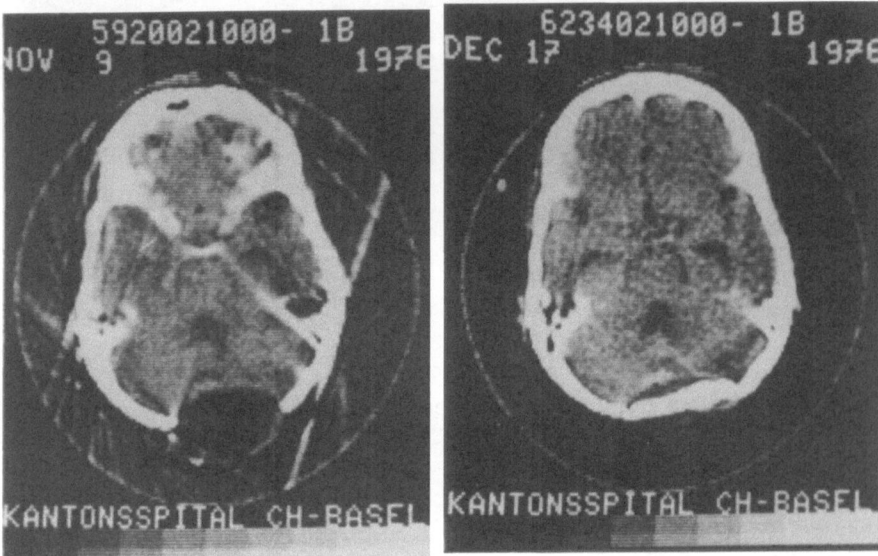

Fig. 41a   Fig. 41b

Fig. 41a. CSF cyst, formed after the removal of a traumatic subdural haematoma of the posterior cranial fossa

Fig. 41b. Condition after cranioplasty with Palacos® R

3. Protection Against Mechanical Influences

In children, in patients with existing minimal brain disorder or with epileptic fits as well as in head-injured patients of special professions (car mechanics, drivers, policemen etc.), a repair of the skull defect is particularly indicated as protective measure against external mechanical influences. In general, though, in these patients the special danger of injury is not necessarily high [111]. But various protective helmets, specially made for this purpose, are

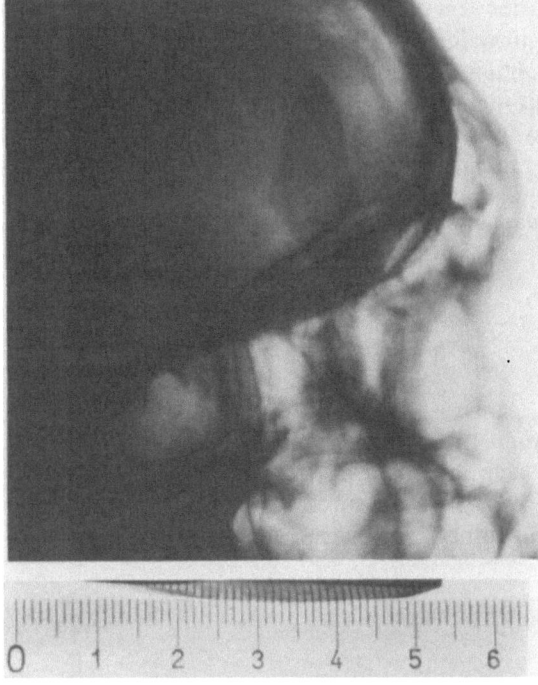

Fig. 42. A 26-year-old schizophrenic thrust a 4 cm long glass splinter through the cranial defect into the cranium. The bone defect in the right frontal region was caused by an earlier suicidal attempt with a revolver

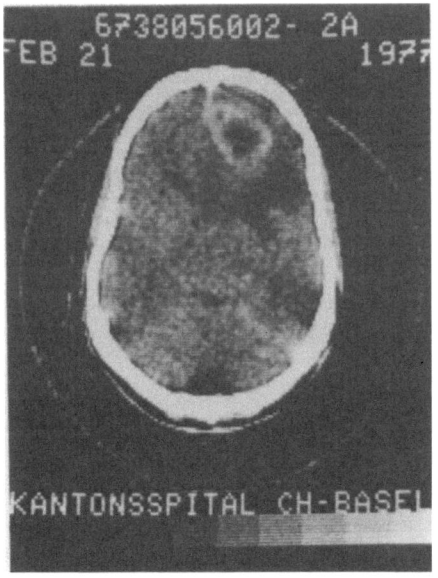

Fig. 43. A brain abscess developed in the right frontal region 2 months later

often a heavy burden for the patient, especially in the hot season; moreover, they are not practical in every profession [158].

Sometimes, patients with posttraumatic brain damage syndromes, depression or other psychic disturbances have to be surgically treated because of attempted suicide by various objects such as needles, nails, screwdrivers, glass splinters, or even matches which have been introduced into the bone defect. In 3 (1.4%) of our patients this was the primary reason for covering the cranial defect. It is noteworthy that, for instance, one young schizophrenic patient developed a brain abscess after she pushed glass splinters into the bone defect (Figs. 42 and 43).

4. Cosmetic Restoration

There is no doubt that a large cranial defect is disfiguring to a high extent. In everyday life, such patients are severely handicapped by comparison to the healthy persons, especially because laymen have the tendency to deduce exaggerated implications from every even harmless injury [145]. These facts

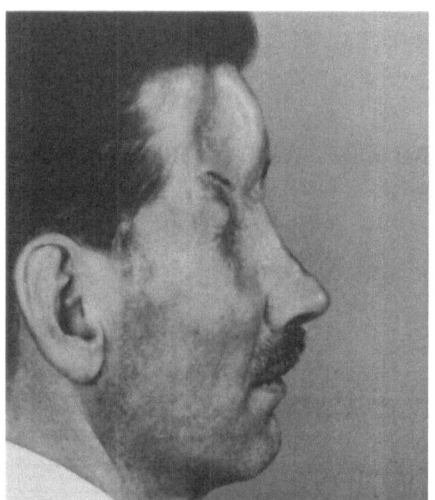 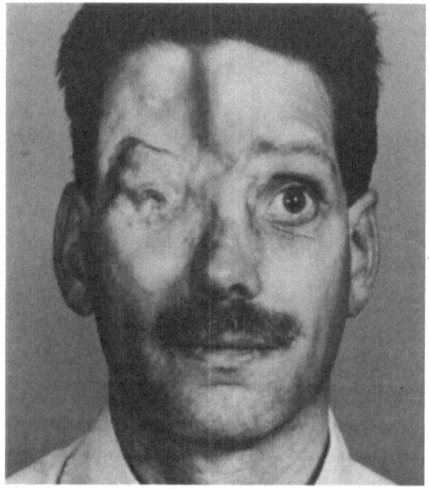

Fig. 44. Severe open craniocerebral injury of the right fronto-basal region caused 12 years before by an explosion. Large defect of the right frontal bone with blindness

represent serious social and psychic problems for the patient, in particular when a very deforming and clearly visible bone defect exists as for instance on the forehead [67, 111]. Not to forget are the difficulties in obtaining work or the continuous psychological frustration to which the patient is exposed through the pitying or inquisitive glaring of his surrounding. Moreover, these patients are harrassed by constant anxiety of possible injury of the unprotected brain (Fig. 44). Altogether, the problems encountered in such situations, are

manyfold and cannot be easily overcome [145]. Correctly performed cranioplasty, which restores the normal proportions of the head and face (Fig. 45), is
a cosmetic measure, but with profound consequences in respect to the affective
and social life of the patients [107, 160].

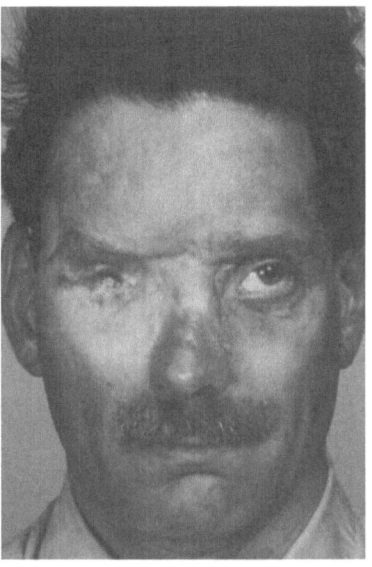

Fig. 45. The same patient as in Fig. 44, 6 months after cranioplasty (Palacos® R with
Gentamycin). Before long, an artificial eye will be prepared by the ophthalmologist

II. Contraindications

There are not very many contraindications for performing cranioplasty.
They could be divided into five groups:

1. raised intracranial pressure and brain prolapse,
2. skin necrosis with consecutive defects,
3. local and generalized infections,
4. cranial defects with communication to the paranasal sinus (only for cranioplasty with acrylates)* and
5. small bone defects (diameter less than 2 cm) which are covered with a layer
   of thick muscle.

---

* It should be stressed, however, that since the appearance of acrylates combined with
antibiotics, providing also that appropriate surgical technique is applied, this contraindication has
lost topical interest.

1. Raised Intracranial Pressure and Brain Prolapse

A decompressive craniotomy must be attempted as ultimate possibility [96], especially when a severe postcontusional ("malignant") brain oedema with brain mass displacement does not respond to the conventional osmo- or, the newer, barbiturate therapy [181]. This may happen after removal of an acute subdural or intracerebral haematoma with progressive brain stem compression. Under such circumstances, besides craniotomy, enlargement of

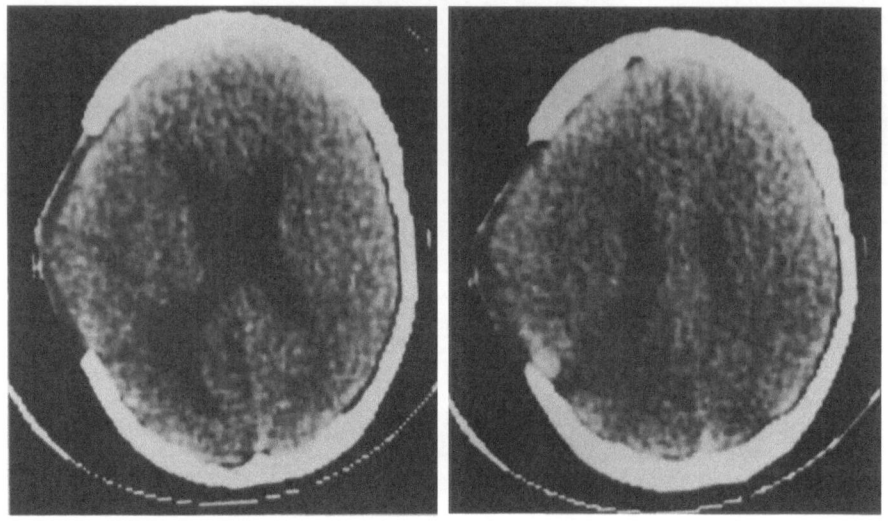

Fig. 46a   Fig. 46b

Fig. 46a, b. A 25-year-old patient with severe contusio cerebri, 3 weeks after decompression because of an oedema, untreatable by drug therapy. Brain prolapse is still present

the dura (with muscle, galea, lyophilized dura of fascia lata) plays an essential role in the expansion of the brain. As a result of the decompression, a brain prolapse evolves through the bone defect and could remain so for several weeks. Decompressive trepanation of this type was performed in 36% of our patients. An illustrative case is presented in Fig. 46 (a, b).

A cranioplasty, undertaken under such conditions (with raised intracranial pressure) would not have the desired effect.

A bone lid or acrylate prosthesis inserted under pressure can cause the already existing intracranial pressure to further increase. The closure of the cranial defect cannot be performed, unless the intracranial pressure has stabilized and the brain prolapse regressed. In our experience, for optimal cranioplasty at least 3 months after the stabilization should expire [159].

2. *Skin Necrosis*

The state of the skin flap overlying the defect is an important factor in cranioplasty. The latter is contraindicated in cases of skin necrosis and skin defects, especially for heteroplastic closures. After craniocerebral injuries, where the scalp is also damaged and postoperatively poorly vascularized as

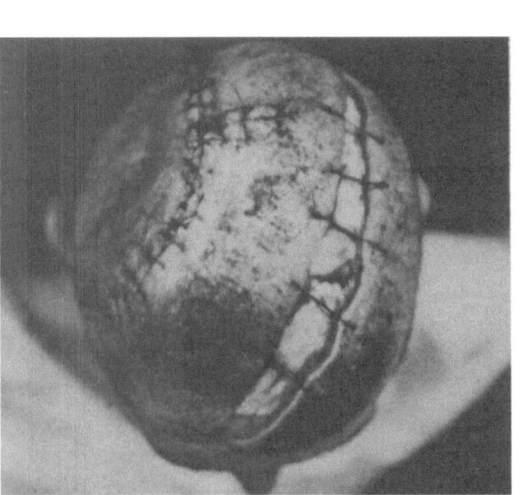
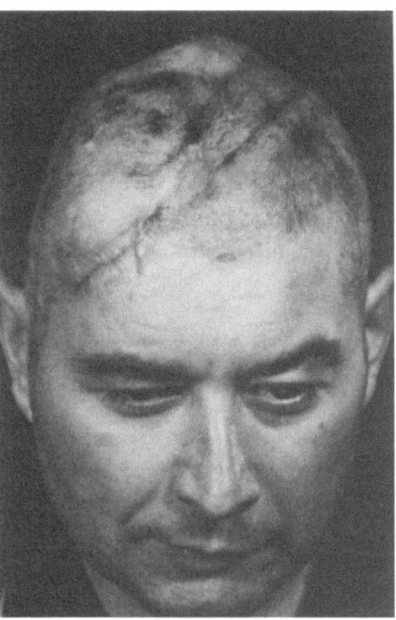

Fig. 47   Fig. 48

Fig. 47. A 37-year-old patient after repeated operations for a recurrent malignant convexity meningioma. A cranioplasty was performed with Palacos® R. The large skin defect was covered by a sliding flap and a Thiersch's graft. Condition 1 week postoperatively

Fig. 48. The same patient as in Fig. 47, 6 weeks later

well as repeatedly scarred, it is advisable to wait before performing surgical repair. Skin necrosis usually develops under such conditions within a short time, which then requires the removal of the plastic. In such cases it is advisable to carry out "flap-training" [122].

The proposed skin flap is freed from the dura and the bone edges with maximum care. Then, the skin flap is replaced into the same position and fixed only with adaption sutures. A plastic closure could be undertaken subsequently, when after a week the skin shows no circulatory disturbances. This procedure has proved useful in such cases and has been repeatedly applied.

Large scalp defects originating from malignant tumours, burns or injuries, represent a serious problem in reconstructive cranial surgery. The attempts have been made to solve this problem by means of a sliding flap, alone or combined with a Thiersch's graft [26] as illustrated in Figs. 47 and 48, which, however, did not always result in an aesthetic success. Recently, there is an increasing number of reports showing successful plastic coverage of large skin defects with free skin flap grafts [45, 88], using microsurgical technique. According to these reports – we have not been able to collect any experience of our own so far – this method appears to be promising.

3. Localized and General Infections

Skin infection like pyodermia or infections which appear especially in open craniocerebral injuries, and also not too seldom in closed injuries, represent another contraindication for cranioplasty. Purulent fistulae lying in the region of the skin cicatrices, various ceragranulomas, non-absorbed sutures and small

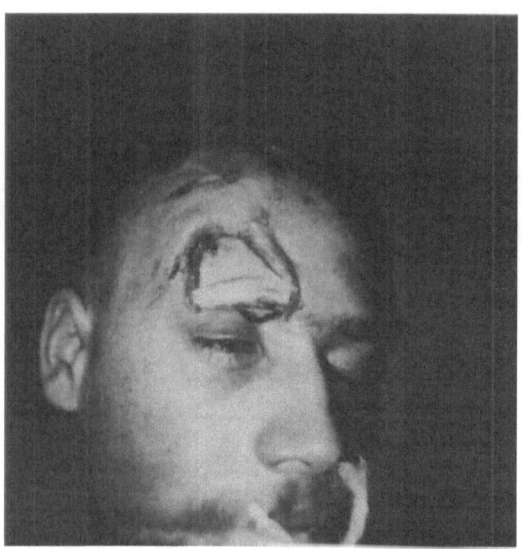

Fig. 49. Wound infection with widespread skin necrosis after cranioplasty with Palacos® R following open craniocerebral injury. Condition after 2 months

retained bone fragments, which are often contaminated with staphylococci, usually do not heal spontaneously. Such an infection can be eliminated only by a surgical revision of the wound. According to our experience, antibiotics alone do not have any decisive influence upon such infections. Only about a year after the infection is fully cleaned up and the wound shows no more signs of irritation, cranioplasty could be taken into consideration [71, 74, 79, 160, 165].

Implantation of a foreign body, which is indeed cranioplasty, is of course contraindicated in general infections and septic conditions. The further treatment depends on the condition of the patient and of the infection, and the rule is, the more time elapses after the infection, the less complicated is the postoperative progress (Fig. 49).

4. Cranial Defects with Communication to Paranasal Sinus

The repair of skull defects (by means of acrylates) with open paranasal sinuses was until recently contraindicated because of the danger of infection [6, 74, 141]. Today this condition represents only relative contraindication since new forms of methylmethacrylates into which antibiotics are incorporated (Palacos® R with Gentamycin®, Schering; Riphocim-Palacos® R, Merck) have appeared [87, 133]. It was demonstrated that the antibiotics are released from the methylmethacrylate in a therapeutically effective dosage. Consequently they can act in the immediate surroundings of the acrylate. *In-vitro* studies showed that the relasing process lasts for over 2 or 3 years [17, 175, 176]. Due to these properties, methylmetacrylate with the addition of antibiotics appeared as to provide a prophylaxis against infection, especially in the open impression fractures with a damage of the paranasal sinuses [97].

Some authors [71], however, are strictly against cranioplasty where no radical cleaning-up and atrophy of the open paranasal sinuses has taken place, at least one year before the final defect closure. For the closure of the open paranasal sinuses, a periosteum flap or a free graft was claimed to be necessary before the final layer of the methylmethacrylate plate is inserted [179].

Of 122 of our patients who received an acrylate cranioplasty, 9 (7.3%) were patients with skull defects and open paranasal sinuses. We performed the cranioplasty with Palacos® R with Gentamycin®. All these patients suffered from infections because of the retention of infected secretion in the paranasal sinuses which was in contact with Palacos® R. Nevertheless, we believe that a cranioplasty with acrylates could also be performed in the case of open paranasal sinuses, provided that a rhinosurgical toilet, including optimal drainage of the sinus secretion, is performed beforehand. The appropriate time for this treatment depends on the general condition of the patient and should, where possible, be undertaken at the same time as the cranioplasty [133].

5. Small Cranial Defects

Small cranial defects with a diameter of 2–3 cm must not necessarily be repaired [169]. Usually, there is no reason to operate these defects, especially when they are covered with thick layers of muscle [79]. This situation must not be interpreted, however, as an absolute contraindication. Defects in the region of the forehead, in spite of the small surface area, should be repaired if indicated by cosmetic reasons [159]. The reconstructive surgery is, for instance, especially indicated in patients engaged in public life and, in consequence, continuously exposed to the public (booking clerks, teachers, actors, policemen etc.). Examples of such repairing effect are illustrated in Figs. 50a, b.

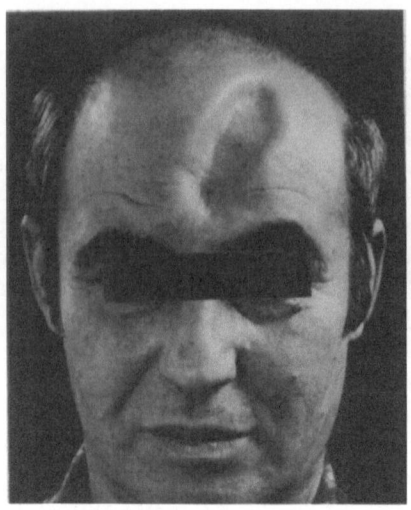 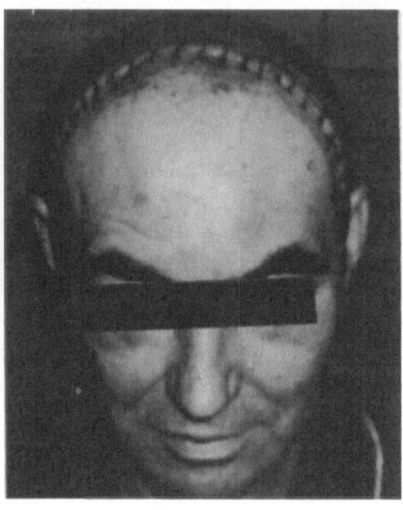

Fig. 50a   Fig. 50b

Fig. 50a. Left-frontal defect after open craniocerebral injury

Fig. 50b. The same patient as in Fig. 50a, 2 days after cranioplasty with Palacos® R with Gentamycin

III. Material Used for Cranioplasty

As can be expected, in the course of time a variety of materials has been used to repair cranial defects [1, 9, 11, 13, 20, 24, 34, 36, 41, 46, 59]. These materials included homologous and heterologous bone grafts, metals and acrylates. For an optimal cranioplasty, it is required that the used materials possess following properties [15, 78]:

1. tissue tolerance,
2. simple manufacturing technique,
3. easy to sterilize,
4. low thermal conductivity,
5. radiolucency and
6. low costs.

Practically none of the available materials entirely fulfills all these demands [16], and for that reason the choice of material is rather large [15, 71, 152]:

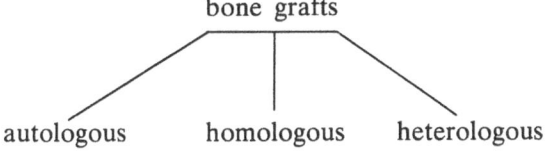

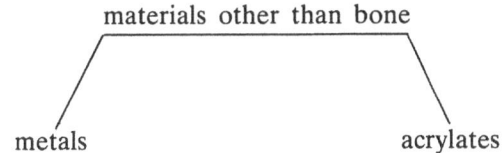

1. Bone Grafts

1.1 Autologous Grafts

1.1.1 Periosteum-Bone Flap Taken from the Vicinity of the Cranial Bone Defect

A periosteum-bone flap for cranioplasty of small defects was first used by Müller in 1890. Since then this method has been repeatedly modified and improved [94].

The bone defect is laid open through a pedicled skin flap. Then a pedicled periosteum flap is cut out alongside of the defect, and the piece of bone corresponding to the size of the defect is carved out with a sharp chisel. The newly formed periosteum bone flap is moved over on its pedicle to cover the bone defect and fixed with sutures to the surrounding periosteum (von Hacker–Durante modification, Fig. 51).

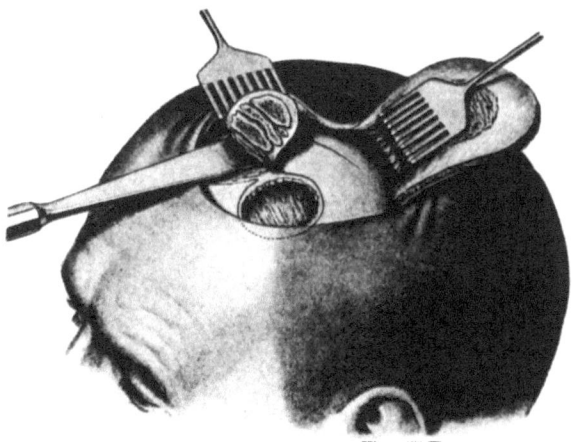

Fig. 51. Cranioplasty according to von Hacker–Durante

1.1.2 Tibial Grafts

The tibial periosteum-graft introduced by Seydel in 1889 was used for a number of years on small defects with mostly good results. Disadvantages are the small surface area from where the graft is removed, the lack of the specific calotte contour of the chip and the resulting tibia fractures [111]. Apart from that, two operations are necessary, and in the postoperative phase many patients complain more of pain in their legs than in the head [8]. With the progress achieved in the technique of cranioplasty and the discovery of new materials this procedure is only of historical interest.

1.1.3 Rib Grafts

First reports about closures of skull defects with autologous rib ("split rib graft") appeared in 1915 [91, 100]. In the beginning, the whole thickness of the rib with the periosteum was used; later on, however, it was preferred to split the rib [6] without considerably reducing the strength of the graft. The inner portion of the rib remained in the patient as protection for the contents of the thorax.

It was certainly an advantage to win a whole graft area which made the closure of large defects possible. Ribs regenerate quickly and can, therefore, be used again for grafting at a later date (the inexhaustible autologous bone bank). This material is characterized by its flexibility and can be as well easily formed with a scalpel. It is especially suitable in the reconstruction of the profile of the supra-orbital curve [117]. Apart from good bony union at the edge of the graft, the formation of an osseous bridge between the gaps of the rib graft follows within a short time [128]. In spite of numerous biological and technical advantages, this method, however, failed to receive any general consideration. The reason is, as in every graft with autologous bone, presumably the necessity of a second operation.

1.1.4 Iliac Crest Grafts

This method was also developed during World War I. In adults, a large piece of bone up to 10×20 cm^2 can be obtained [147]. The advantage of this method is that it provides a large concave–convex graft, similar in form to that of the skull. As a consequence, a good cosmetic result, especially in the frontal region, could be achieved. The considerable length of the surgical procedure, which implicates quite a heavy blood loss due to the muscularity of this area as well as the later growth problem in children, are marked disadvantages of this method. Nevertheless, in the reconstructive surgery today it is still advocated that bone from this source gives a reliable and satisfactory tissue for cranioplasty.

1.1.5 Scapula and Sternum Grafts

Autologous scapula grafts were first used at the beginning of World War I [143]. These grafts are not used any more, although they have certain advantages, such as for example periosteum from both sides and a natural convexity.

1.1.6 Cartilage Grafts

This method became known during World War I. Several skull defects were covered with cartilage taken from ribs of patients [25, 134]. This method was accepted enthusiastically at the beginning of the 1920's, as cartilage is easy to model and resistant to infection. Conserved autologous and homologous cartilage was also used to repair defects, especially those of the small supra-orbital region. This method has been discontinued in the last years because of its complicated procedure.

1.2 Homologous Grafts

Cranial bone removed from living patients or corpses is used for homologous grafts [71, 118, 149]. The bony material is taken from craniotomy patients who for various reasons could not have the bone reimplanted. The removed material is usually conserved in a bone bank and then later implanted into another patient [146]. In a so-called parallel procedure, still vital bone from the patient can be implanted into another already prepared patient (Figs. 52a, b).

The advantage of this procedure lies in the possibility of being able to immediately implant healthy and sterile bone without using conservation [9]. We used this method in two patients. Four years after grafting we were able to see at the macroscopic level perfect bone consolidation in both of the implants. Skull bone removed under sterile conditions from corpses can also be used directly or after conservation in the bone bank for implants. This method was suggested by Ollier, who obtained "transplantation material" from amputated extremities of war-injured soldiers and used it immediately for implantation into other patients (for ref. see [146]).

Over 120 cases with very satisfactory results were reported between 1917 and 1919 from a number of authors who used bone for cranioplasty from autopsy cases. In an article in 1947 on plastic closure of skull defects, Bushe concluded that homologous bone could be used for grafting under the same circumstances as autologous bone (for ref. see [146]).

The theoretical basis for using foreign bone is the autogenetic fact that cranial bone is derived from connective tissue and can be substituted [62, 63, 118, 150]. As the osteogenetic substance of the transplants becomes destroyed, implants function only as conductors and are replaced by a creeping substitution by own body bone coming from the margin of the defect. In an implant of some 5 cm in diameter this takes approximately 2 years [107, 166]. Apart from the fact that the use of cadaver bone [118] presents a somewhat disquieting method, the procedure fell into disfavour after numerous reports of rejection and infection [69].

1.3 Heterologous Grafts

Long ago, the closure of skull defects was reputed to be the classical domain of xenogeneic grafting [174], but nowadays it has little more than

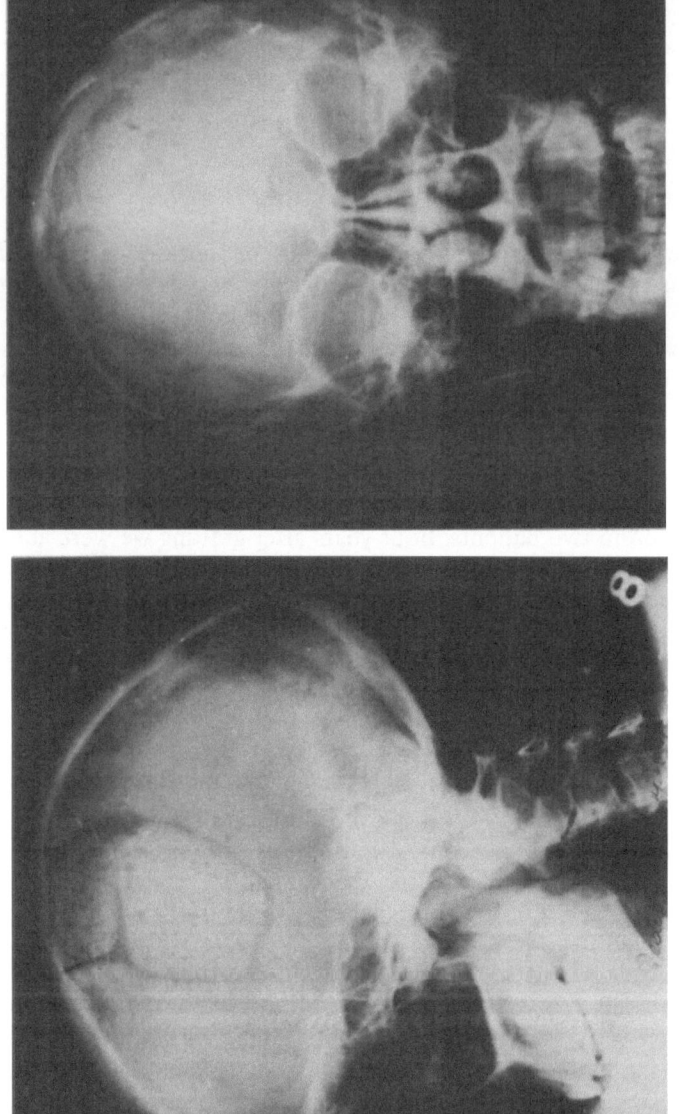

Fig. 52a

Fig. 52b

Fig. 52a, b. A "parallel procedure" was performed on a 30-year-old patient with left parietal, open craniocerebral injuries. Part of the cranial bone of another seriously injured patient who died intra-operatively, was implanted. The X-rays were taken 6 months postoperatively

historical interest. Occasionally, it was performed with oxen-horn plates, sometimes with success [24, 107]. In most cases, however, the grafts were resorbed or rejected.

2. Materials Other than Bone

2.1 Metals

In 1565, Petronius undertook the first attempt of cranioplastic closure with a gold plate [109, 137, 171, 174]. More than three hundred years later (1893), cranioplasty was again tried using another metal, aluminium [11]. Gold, silver and even lead were used during a certain period of time at the beginning of the twentieth century [90]. During and after World War II, especially some authors favoured the use of tantalum [44, 49, 178], ticonium [22] or vitalium plates [22, 135] for cranioplasty. Stainless steel was also applied [52, 152]. These metals had to be hammered into shape, which did not always produce the desired cosmetic result. The foreign body irritation caused granulation tissue, formation of fistulae, sequestration and other complications [2, 137, 174].

Disadvantages of these materials are the difficulty to model, impermeability to X-rays, corrosion to a certain extent (silver oxide), symptoms of intoxication (lead) and necrosis [1, 174]. On the other hand, a single surgical intervention, low costs and a practically unlimited source of material available can be quoted as advantages.

2.2 Acrylates

Acrylates found little consideration in reconstructive cranial surgery after Fraenkel's [48] attempt in 1894 to close a skull defect with celluloid, as Kleinschmitt could demonstrate that celluloid possessed tissue irritating, possibly cancerogenic properties [93]. The year 1939 witnessed a rebirth of acrylate material. At that time polymethacrylate, called plexiglass, which was compatible with the connective tissue, was discovered [13, 46, 85, 89, 94]. After World War II, paladon (plexiglass-polymerizate), palavit and recently palacos were developed. At the moment, acrylates of this type represent the most appropriate alloplastic material for cranioplasty [41, 71, 79, 140, 159, 173, 180] and are applied either in the monomeric (liquid) or polymeric (powder) form. The paste formed by both components hardens by a polymerization process [17, 36, 169].

They are available as warm-polymerizing (polymerization occurs slowly by application of heat and pressure) and as cold-polymerizing (polymerization occurs quickly by chemical energy) acrylates [13, 107]. The cold-polymerizing methylacrylates imply, however, a certain danger of thermonecrosis at the implantation site, due to high polmerization temperatures [28, 82]. Measurements with an avoidance of direct contact with the hardening bone cement, by means of infra-red thermography, showed polymerization temperatures of over 100 °C [82] which coincides with our measurements using direct methods (Fig. 53).

Irrespectively of the size of the bone cement piece, we found equal temperatures of over 100 °C. We could confirm that heat production during polymerization of the cement tested did not depend on the ratio of surface area to the volume [82]. The average hardening time varies, depending on the type of cement used, between 1 and 12 minutes. All methylacrylates reach high temperatures, far above the albumin coagulation temperature of 56 °C as reported by Lehnartz [113].

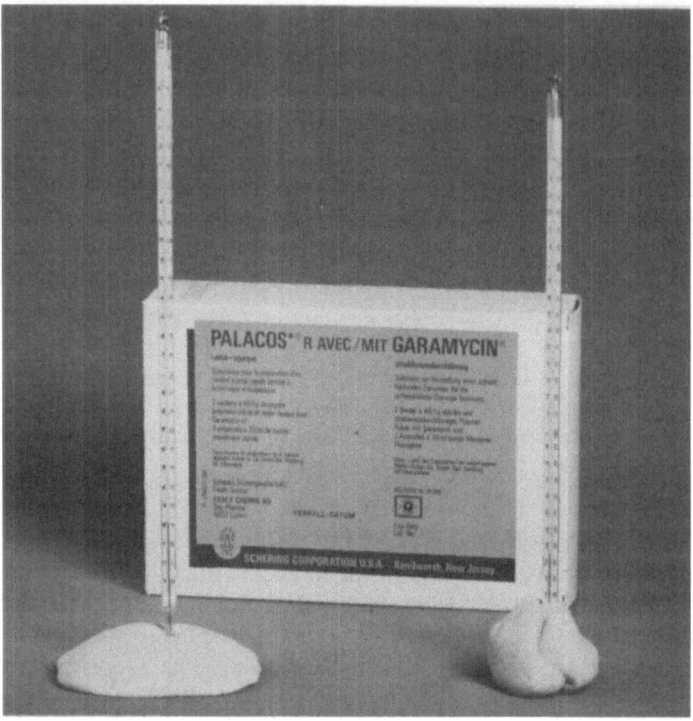

Fig. 53. Direct measurement of the temperature of two similar sized, but differently modelled pieces of resin

The powder of quick-hardening acrylates (bone cements) is supplied in several commercial forms: Palacos® R, Bone cement®, Riphocim-Palacos® R, Palacos® R with Garamycin® R (Gentamycine) in Europe and Simplex* (Howmedica) L.V.C.® and Bone Cement® (Zimmer) in U.S.A.

The advantage of cold-polymerizing acrylates lies in the possibility of modelling directly during the operation as well as the fast and technically simple production of the required acrylate object. The amount of residual monomers which are liberated in these acrylates is, according to recent tests, too small to have any cytotoxic effects [77].

Warm-polymerizing acrylates contain practically no residual monomer; preparation of an implant is, however, more complicated than by

---

* Surgical Simplex® P (radiopaque bone cement) and Surgical Simplex® P (bone cement).

"cold"-polymerizing cements [16, 36]. A wax or plaster model of the skull defect is taken, the acrylate is cast according to the prepared model and then sent to a specially equipped laboratory for polymerization which takes approximately 24 hours [1, 173]. Only after sterilization the prosthesis is ready for implantation. Besides a minimum output of residual monomer, an essential advantage of a lengthy polymerization process is that the implant can be carefully planned without haste, then produced, and the appointed operating date can be fixed to suit the time requirements [36].

IV. Conservation Procedures

1. The Problem of Bone Graft Conservation

It is necessary to store the bone pieces for a certain period of time if they are not immediately needed. Current autoplastic bone grafting is known to be connected with some disadvantage, since to remove a bone chip and implant in the same operation, means an extra risk, as it lengthens the procedure. In addition, the patients are burdened with an additional bone defect which often regenerates slowly and incompletely [146].

The idea of conserving bone is old. In the first half of the twentieth century the transplantation of fresh bone tissue was somewhat neglected, whereas the problem of bone conservation again received much interest as a consequence of the doctrine of Bart, who claimed the equivalence of fresh living and dead bone [5].

2. Methods of Conservation

The oldest conservation methods of boiling in water or storage in alcohol and mercury have been maintained here and there up until today [146, 174]. However, boiling and macerating the bone was never fully satisfactory as a method of conservation. Boiling destroys the osteogenetic potential of the bone chip and furthermore, the tendency of infection and absorption is increased [146].

2.1 Deep Freezing

The successful conservation of food by deep freezing encouraged the attempt to use the same method for tissues and organs needed for transplantation [21]. The first bone bank was opened by L. F. Bush in 1945 in the Orthopaedic Hospital in New York [146]. There are, however, a few problems connected to the deep freezing procedure. Firstly, a perfect supervision service of the bone bank must exist, which increases the costs, and secondly a temperature of -20 to $-25\,°C$, which is generally necessary for good conservation, must continuously be maintained.

In the last few years more and more cases of osteolysis of reimplanted cranial bone conserved by deep freezing have been reported [34]. This compares with our own experiences. In a total of 84 of our patients with cranioplasty carried out with a graft from the bone bank, 59 patients (70%) showed signs of absorption two years after the surgery.

2.2 Conservation of the Cranial Bone Under the Abdominal Wall

Immediately after World War I (1920) and shortly before the introduction of conservation by low temperatures, a new method began to be tested [70, 83, 84]. Several cranial bone fragments were removed from a five year old boy

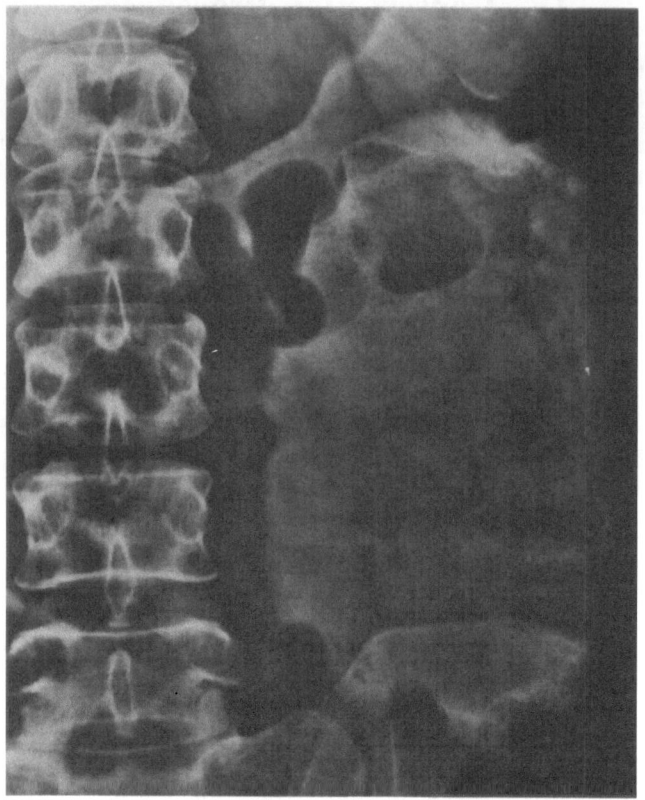

Fig. 54. X-ray: Bone in left upper abdomen 4 weeks after implantation

after an open brain injury and implanted under the abdominal wall of the patient. The bone was removed approximately 3 months later without complication and reimplanted into the skull defect [103]. The case of conservation of the bone in the abdominal wall is illustrated in Fig. 54.

It should be noted that the right abdominal side is not recommended for conservation in the case an eventual appendix operation is necessary. The bone graft is placed into a prepared pocket in the left upper abdomen so that its

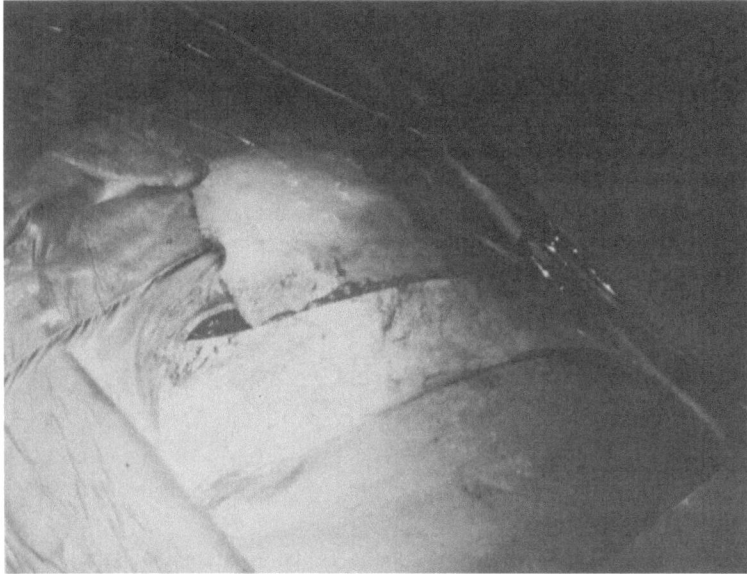

Fig. 55. The bone graft was taken out during a decompression craniotomy for the removal of an acute subdural haematoma and implanted in the abdominal wall

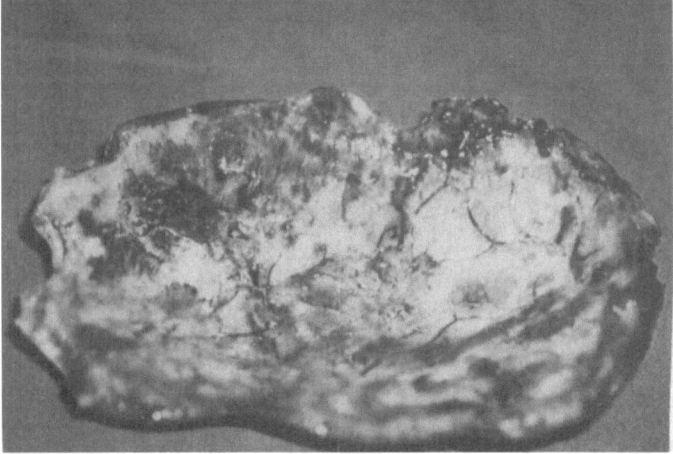

Fig. 56. The bone graft removed from the abdomen after 3 months of implantation shows macroscopic vitality signs. Nevertheless the bone margin shows marked signs of resorption

curvature fits into the abdominal contours. A redivac drain is inserted and the skin closed with deep sitting sutures (Fig. 55).

The bone graft which is removed from the abdominal wall after about 3 months shows thin macroscopic signs of living bone (Fig. 56).

Autologous, cancellous bone grafts in a rabbit, conserved in a similar fashion, also showed signs of regeneration [70, 103, 153]. Although this method of storing and conserving skull bones fulfills all requirements for an optimal cranioplasty – the patient's own bone, sterile tissue (abdominal wall) serves as a bone storage place, and the vitality of the bone is partially retained – the method is not widely used. The development of other conservation procedures has led this process to be abandoned. Nevertheless, as practically all conservation techniques have more than one drawback, it is worthwhile to describe here this nearly forgotten method of placing the implant under the abdominal wall. The advantages and disadvantages of this procedure are summarized in Table 8.

Table 8. *Advantages and Disadvantages of Conserving Bone Under the Abdominal Wall*

Advantages	Disadvantages
no bone bank necessary – temperature and sterility controls can therefore be omitted	two operations are necessary
partial retainment of the vitality of the bone	a large abdominal scar
optimal cosmetic result	large bone pieces cause a pressure when carried and give an unpleasant feeling when bending
quick and inexpensive operation	
independence of the patient: the bone can be reimplanted in any hospital	

Casuistic

In 10 patients with an acute subdural haematoma, a decompressive trepanation was performed after haematoma removal, and the removed bone was placed under the abdominal wall. The oldest patient was 72 years old, the youngest 17 years old. Four patients died of their injuries a few days postoperatively, but 6 recovered quite well. The first bone reimplantation was carried out in a conventional way, about one month after the accident. The bone removed from the abdominal wall and implanted in the cranial defect showed macroscopic signs of vitality, but also some resorption changes on the bone edge. These were also found in 5 other reimplantations which we performed 2–6 months after the accident. A postoperative check-up a year later showed no new resorption signs. The wounds showed non-irritated, p.p. healing, and we saw only one infected wound in a patient who died of his injuries.

By comparing pathophysiological findings with deep frozen cranial bone, which after 3 months showed complete necrosis of osteocytes and myeloid tissue, the bone graft after 3 months in the abdominal wall showed besides areas of necrosis new metaplastic bone formation. In the following, short descriptions of the pathohistology of the bones from the abdominal walls in two patients are given.

1st Patient E-No 8022/80 (17 years old)

Biopsy of skull bone (3 times), condition during 6 weeks after implantation under the abdominal wall. Vascularization? Three greyish-white, mainly compact, partly cancellous bone fragments, measuring together 15 mm in max. ∅.

Histological diagnosis:

Parts of skull bone with complete necrosis as well as a large penetration of the diploë spaces by angiofibrous myeloid tissue, *focal formation of new fibrous bone trabeculae* free in myeloid tissue as well as in connection with dead bone.

2nd Patient E-No 7704-05/80 (60 years old)

Cranial bone from abdominal wall (3 months after implantation). Histological parts of compact bone with wide cancellous spaces which are filled with vital fibrous connective tissue. Here and there wide sinus type capillaries are present. In one place there is a *formation of metaplastic new bone* in the connective tissue to a small extent. The old bone shows only empty osteocyte formation.

(Extracts from original reports of histological examinations of skull bone deposited under the abdominal wall before reimplantation in patients; Institute of Pathology, Medical Faculty of University of Basle.)

V. Operative Technique

1. General Considerations

Before admission to hospital, every patient showing an indication for cranioplasty is first clinically examined. The following points are paid attention to:

1. condition of the operating area, especially the cicatrice of the craniotomy,
2. neurological status,
3. general condition,
4. age and profession.

Furthermore, helped by case histories and autoanamnesis, the interval between the craniotomy or last reoperation is determined, and the existence of any bone or skin infections is also reviewed. Depending on these factors, the urgency of the operation is determined and the operating plan set up. Whether the cranioplasty is to be performed with the patient's own bone or foreign bone or with alloplastic material depends on several factors: the condition of the patient's own bone, the size and localization of the cranial defect, and the distance from the paranasal sinuses. The patient is usually admitted to hospital one day before the operation so that skull X-rays and computer tomography (CT) can be made in order to detect possible brain tissue displacements, porencephalic cysts, hydrocephalus internus, or a space occupying lesion (e.g. abscess). The head is completely shaved on the day of the operation and the scalp again carefully examined.

1.1 Flap Formation

A p.p. linear scar overlying the defect may be utilized again. When the scar is star-shaped or otherwise irregular it is advisable to avoid reusing it for the incision and to plan a skin flap sufficiently distant from the defect to ensure adequate blood supply and uneventful healing [59, 86].

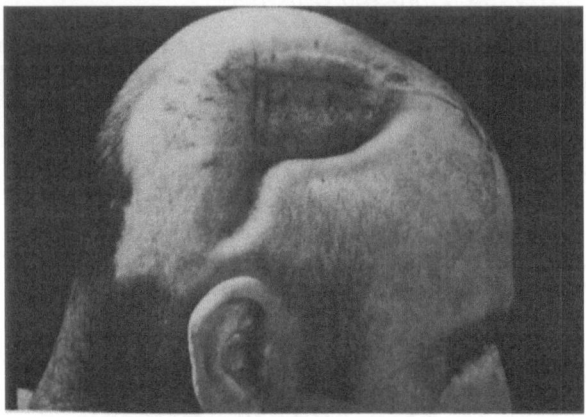

Fig. 57. A 42-year-old patient after open craniocerebral injuries. The well-healed scar can be again used for cranioplasty

In order to avoid possible contamination of the new skin incision, the operation wound is again examined carefully for the presence of retained sutures. Suture material which protrudes out of the wound is removed, and a local wound toilet is performed.

1.2 Anaesthesia/Position

The operation usually takes place in general anaesthesia with an endotracheal intubation. The patient is so positioned that the place of the skull defect lies horizontal, with all contours of the skull gap visible and accessible. For obvious reasons, this position offers special advantages in alloplastic closures.

1.3 Haemostasis

Haemostasis is carried out in the usual manner when the wound is not made through the old incision. Haemostasis is seldom needed when the old wound with its scar tissue is opened. By all means, sparsely vascularized scar tissue must be protected from additional trauma. Here, the problem of bleeding is often solved by simply covering the area with a moist gauze.

Of essential importance – often the success of the operation entirely depends upon it – is the condition of the skin flap. A thin, scarred and poorly vascularized skin flap receives even less blood after the insertion of the prosthesis, and necrosis is then unavoidable (Fig. 58).

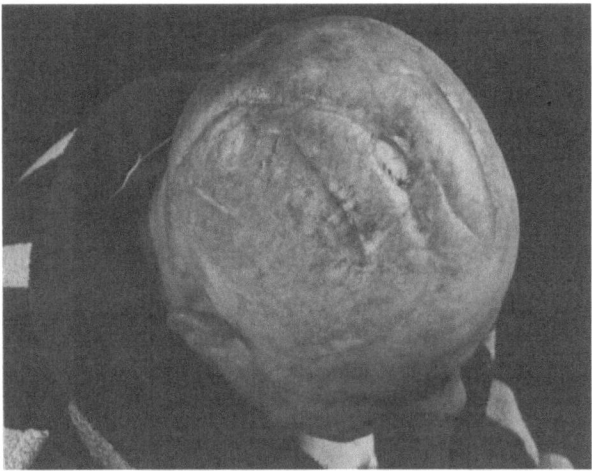

Fig. 58. Skin necrosis after cranioplasty performed with acrylate (Palacos® R) caused by a poorly vascularized skin flap with several scars

2. Operative Procedure

2.1 Preparation of the Skin Flap

The preparation of the skin flap must be carried out in such a way that the scalp retains its original thickness or (through the freeing of adhesions with the dura) becomes even thicker than originally.

The bone edges are prepared until they are completely free [86, 174]. The whole dura surface as well as the inner side of the skin is then carefully inspected. Any existing dura defects or those arising intraoperatively are then well repaired either with sutures or adhesives [64, 121, 144, 157]. Remaining pieces of wax and suspicious granulation must be fully removed and, if necessary, sent for bacteriological examination. In the case of a questionable infection, it is better to terminate the operation at this stage and await bacteriological results, than to undertake a plastic closure with an unsure outcome [108]. The so prepared operating field is then abundantly rinsed with antiseptic Polybactrin* Solubile or Betadine** Solution Antiseptique [12].

---

* Polybactrin Solubile: Polymyxin-B-sulfat, Bacitracin, Neomycinsulfat, WELLCOME.
** Betadine: Solution Antiseptique, Polyvinilpyrrolidonum c 10%, Iodum 10%, MUNDIPHARMA AG.

2.2 Bone Transplant

The bone transplant for the plastic is removed from the bone bank about one hour before implantation and soaked in an antibiotic (Penicillin) solution until needed.

The fixation with Kirschner's wires or wire loops, as was earlier performed, is not used anymore, as patients often complained of pain over the fixation area, and it was not unusual to observe skin perforation. As well, the practice of drilling small holes in the skull bone (to allow drainage of exsudate) has been disregarded. Our experience and that of other authors shows that the multiple perforations produce a necrotic focus over a large area and lead to progressive resorption of the skull bone [34, 160], as illustrated in Fig. 59.

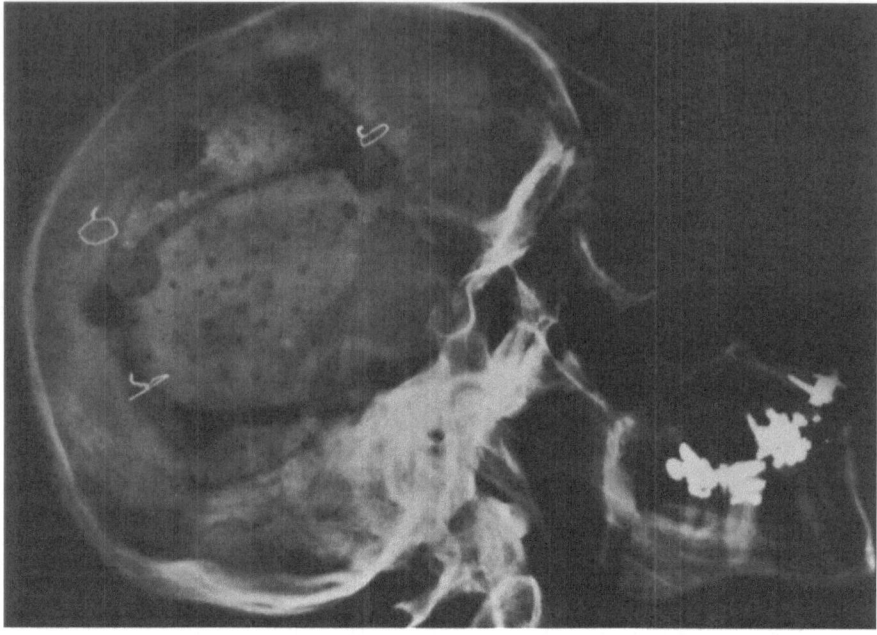

Fig. 59. Patients own bone, partially resorbed, showing multiple perforations and fixation with wire loops

Before the skull bone is fitted into the defect, at least two sides of the skull bone edge should be freed from any tissue and freshened up. This gives the transplant a larger contact area and promotes an eventual, later revitalization of the transplant [107, 127, 138]. After this the implant is well secured into the skull with at least four non-absorbing merilene sutures. In this method we have observed no slackening in the fixation [159].

An epidural drain is always inserted, and if there is any liquid formation after its removal, it is extracted by puncture.

The same principles are used for the implantation of foreign bone. However, especially difficult is the fitting of the prosthesis into the skull defect, and the procedure is often very time consuming [118, 149]. After termination of the operation, a compression bandage is made and left for at least 48 hours.

2.3 Particular Problems of "Sinking Skin Flap Syndrome"

Large, long-standing cranial defects with already extensive cicatrical changes in epi- and subdural spaces do not usually return to normal spontaneously. Not to recognize this problem can have grave consequences, no matter which material is used for the cranioplasty. A large hollow space which can then fill with blood, seroma or cerebrospinal fluid (CSF) is created between the repaired skull and the incompletely extended dura surface. In the latter case (CSF) this is possibly due to an existing communication with the subarachnoid space through the injured dura, which favours the spread of infection throughout the central nervous system (Fig. 60).

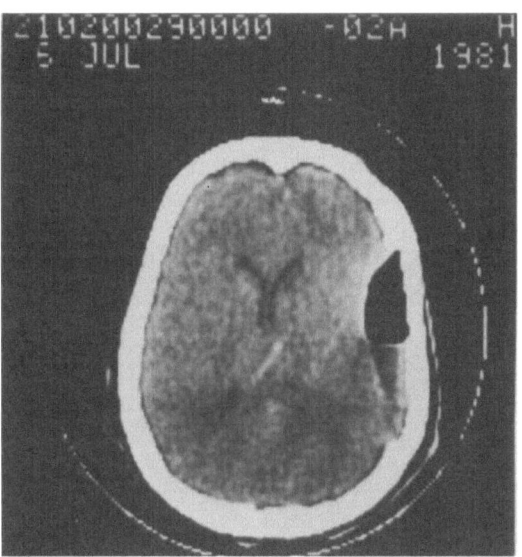

Fig. 60. A 52-year-old patient: cranioplasty with Palacos® R with Gentamycin was performed 11 months after the removal of an acute subdural haematoma. The brain tissue did not expand properly and a haematoma which later became infected, formed in the empty space between the dura and Palacos® plastic

In such situation cranioplasty is not always easy to perform. Practically every plastic closure of a skull defect fails when the brain tissue is not fully expanded or the dura is pitted and sunken-in.

At our clinic each patient was examined by computer tomography immediately after the induction of anaesthesia. The CSF pressure of the

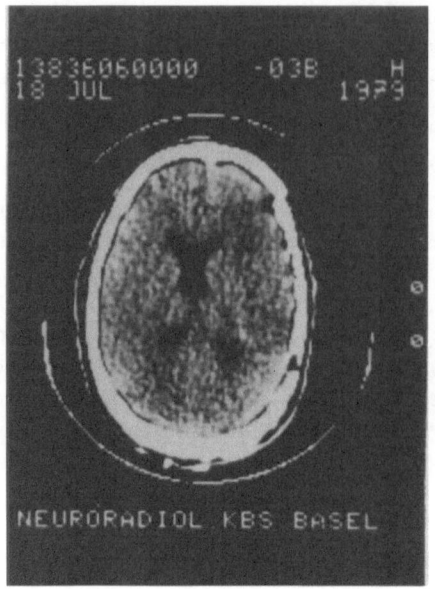
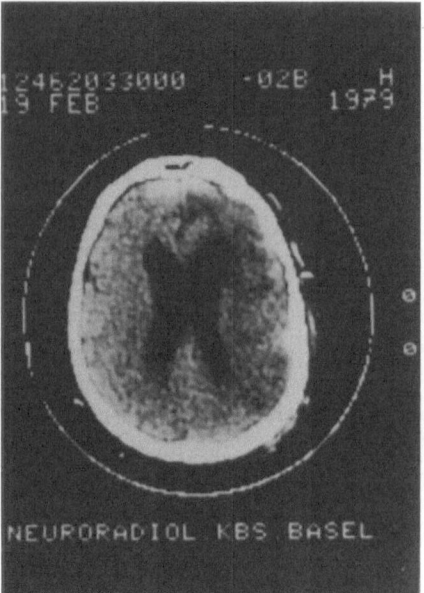

Fig. 61a   Fig. 61b

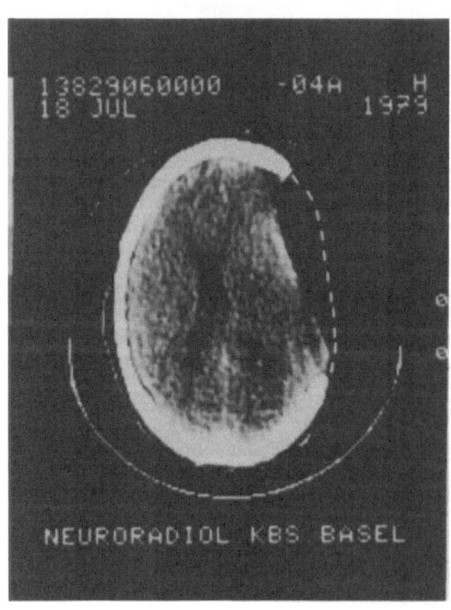
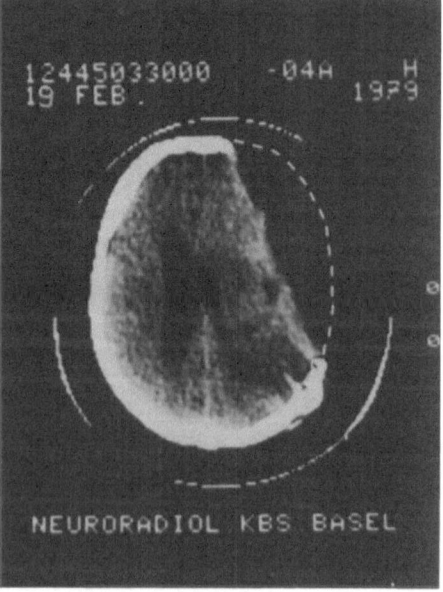

Fig. 62a   Fig. 62b

anaesthetized, recumbent patient was determined by lumbar catheter. All patients had a CSF pressure lower than the normal value of $10-20$ cm H_2O [31, 148]. In four patients aged over 60 years, the pressure varied between 0 and 1 cm H_2O, in three younger patients aged between 30 and 40, the pressure was $2-3$ cm H_2O, and in the three youngest patients (20–30 years), where there were only moderate brain mass displacements, between $6-7$ cm H_2O.

After preparation of the skin flap to allow proper expansion of the brain tissue and to avoid the development of a hollow space between the dura and the cranioplasty, we slowly injected warm (37 °C) physiological saline or Ringer's solution into the subarachnoid space. The injected volume was between $150-180$ ml in patients with a CSF pressure of $0-3$ cm H_2O, and $100-120$ ml in patients with a pressure of $3-6$ cm H_2O. Already during the surgical intervention most patients showed satisfactory expansion of the brain and return of the dura to its normal position.

Some authors have reported this procedure to be dangerous and of no lasting success [116], but in our cases, where we needed a quick intraoperative expansion of the brain, this procedure has proved to be helpful and without risks (Figs. 61a, b).

The main problem in the postoperative progress of the "SSFS" where the intraoperative expansion of the brain is not sufficient, is the formation of a hollow space between the plastic lid and the dura. Here blood, CSF, and serous fluid (seroma) can accumulate (especially in bone cement, cranioplasty) and may become quickly infected (Figs. 62a, b).

An infected haematoma or seroma usually needs an operative revision and the removal of the inserted plastic implant. According to general experience and ours as well, cranioplasty should be repeated only one year later [4, 74, 159]. That means that brain compression and brain mass displacement remain and further influence the general and neurological condition of the patient.

This syndrome and the resulting complications were not always recognized until now. The appropriate procedure, as we introduced it, easily avoids these complications in most cases; the postoperative progress and recovery of the patient can follow without hindrance.

Fig. 61a. Computerized tomography of the skull: A pronounced brain tissue displacement with pitting of the wound appeared in a 46-year-old, anticoagulated patient, some months after removal of an intracerebral haematoma

Fig. 61b. By intraoperative lumbar instillation of Ringer's solution expansion and normalization of the dura is achieved. CT 8 hours postoperatively

Fig. 62a. Condition of a 19-year-old schoolboy 4 months after the removal of an acute subdural haematoma

Fig. 62b. Reversal of the brain mass displacement and normal expansion of the brain occurred intraoperatively after intrathecal administration of saline. CT 10 hours later

3. Cranial Repair Procedure with Bone Transplants

3.1 Homologous Bone

The simplicity of the pretreatment and transplantation of the bone are the reasons why the method, from the technical point of view, could be recommended [9]. The bone material originates from craniotomy patients who for different reasons could have their own bone implanted again.

Before reuse, a bone is selected which corresponds to the size and especially to the bone convexity of the defect. Multiple perforations are drilled in the bone before the implantation. After preparing the operation field in the usual fashion, it is fixed to the surrounding bone with strong, non-absorbing sutures.

The advantage of this method lies in the fact that it can be carried out in every small hospital without any special technical expenditure. However, the use of homologous bone has considerably decreased after the introduction of the bone cements (acrylates) in the reconstructive surgery. Also, a definite disadvantage of the method is a rather high percentage of absorption of the implanted bone.

3.2. Autologous Bone

The bone grafts obtained from the individuals are usually stored in the bone bank, or exceptionally (see below) in the abdominal wall of the patient. The surgical procedure using bone grafts from the bone bank does not greatly differ from the previously described technique. As a rule, the graft should not be inserted earlier than 3 months after the first operation. Under the assumption that the rather high resorption of the bone tissue can be avoided, we have discontinued using bone with multiple perforations. We performed cranial repair with perforated bones in more than half of our patients until 1977, also in order to allow better drainage of the subdural cavity. With non-perforated bone the operating procedure has been simplified, and the duration of surgical procedure has been shortened. A good fixation of the implanted bone to the surrounding calotte bone, good drainage of the operated area, and at least two clean contact sites between the implant and the skull bone are the requirements for a successful operation with this method [98, 131].

Nevertheless, we noticed no clear-cut difference between perforated and non-perforated bone grafts. If anything, somewhat slower resorption of the implant, by comparison to the perforated bone, was noted. The size of the bone graft, the length of the conservation in the bone bank, together with the multiple perforations are suggested to play an important role in the fast resorption of the bone implant [34].

3.2.1 Autologous Bone – Conserved Under the Abdominal Wall

Cranioplasty was carried out in six cases using the patient's own bone which had been "conserved" under the abdominal wall. After the removal of the bone and wound closure, the patient was turned to the dorsal position for the implantation of the skull bone into the abdomen. Then a 10–15 cm long, horizontal skin incision was made in the left epigastrium about 5 cm under the costal margin, and a pocket of the size of the implant was prepared between the skin and the aponeurosis. After the required time (see before) the surgery was performed as described above.

4. Cranial Repair Procedure with Acrylates (Bone Cements)

In the recent years we have repaired cranial defects more and more frequently with bone cements. In the beginning (1968–1975) we used Palacos® R or Bone Cement® without the addition of antibiotic, and since 1975 Riphocim-Palacos® R or Palacos® R with Garamycin® are almost routinely applied. The first phase of the surgical procedure – the preparation of the operative area and the bone defect – does not differ from that mentioned previously. The cranioplasty itself is performed essentially according to the modified Woringer's method [163], with some improvements as recently reported [159, 160]. From the very beginning we have disregarded the pouring of the liquid acrylate into a defect packed with cotton swabs or covered with human amnion, as recommended by some authors [102, 155, 163]. Even when amnion may have the intended function of protecting the wound from chemical damage during the polymerization process, in our opinion this biological insulating material is still not able to provide sufficient protection from the polymerization heat. Apart from this, amnion is difficult to obtain and problematic to sterilize.

Particular disadvantage in the use of quick polymerizing acrylates is the development of the high temperature during the hardening process. As stressed before, several authors carried out tests with the aid of infra-red thermography to measure the polymerization temperature [28, 82, 115]. The resulting average maximum values amounted to 100–120 °C, which is far above the coagulation temperature of 56 °C of albumin, as indicated by Lehnartz [28]. It is, therefore, clear that the polymerization temperature of bone cement can lead to thermonecrosis. It is noteworthy that fatal complications in orthopaedic surgery, where methylmetacrylates were used, have been described [27, 80]. They occurred as a result of an unavoidable and irreversible fall in the blood pressure. Such complications were especially observed in patients with an unstable blood pressure and surgically treated in spinal anaesthesia. Monomers, usually set free during the polymerization of the acrylates, and which enter the blood circulation through the large muscle mass (thigh), were supposed to be the cause of such complications [129].

We found no reports of such severe complications after the use of bone cements in the neurosurgery. Possibly this is due to the smaller amount of acrylates needed to cover the defects and to an operating field which is, by comparison, much less vascularized. In addition, our modification of the procedure of cranioplasty with preparation of the prosthesis not *in situ*, i.e. in the patient, but on the operating table, where the polymerization takes place, also prevents possible transition of the residual monomers into the circulation [159].

Besides that, an additional argument against preparation of the bone cement prosthesis directly onto the bone defect, is the reduced modelling facility of the acrylates under such conditions. The still semi-fluid acrylates mixture which is poured onto the basis of the prepared skull defect, easily assumes the shape of the underlying surface. The resulting form of the prosthesis which is, thus, inadequate, remains definitive after polymerization and hardening [29, 79]. There is no doubt that in the cases of a strongly pitted wound, the functional and aesthetic result obtained by such procedure is unsatisfactory (Fig. 63).

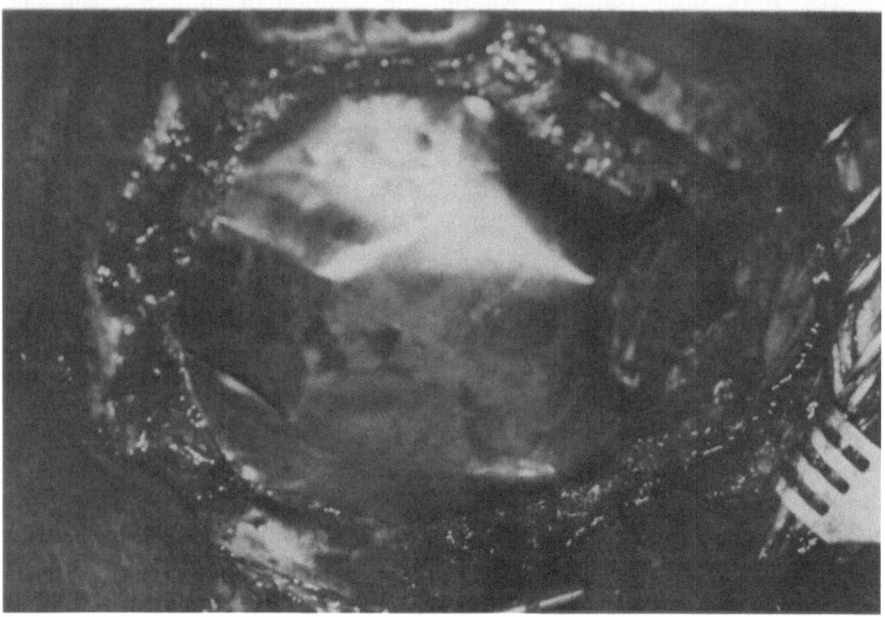

Fig. 63. Modelled zinc plate fitted into the skull defect; a non-polymerized Palacos® mixture is put on the top of it

In the modified bone cement repair procedure, as we applied it, a soft zinc plate is cut to the size of the defect, modelled to the convexity of the skull and then fitted into the gap in the bone. Thereafter, the bone cement powder (polymer) and the liquid part (monomer) are mixed together in a sterile basin in the ratio of 1:1 until a doughy mixture is formed. This mixture is modelled to the thickness of the cranial bone, while still in a soft condition, and then laid over the zinc plate placed over the skull defect. The mass is well fitted into the surrounding bone by means of the finger tips and in such a way as to create a ridgeless junction between the model and the skull bone everywhere. Possible

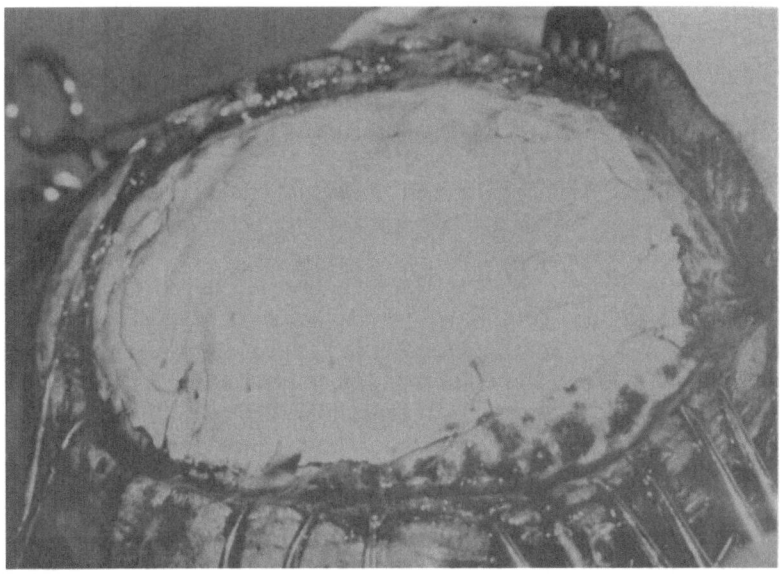

Fig. 64. The bone cement (Palacos®) is cast over the zinc plate. The first phase of the
polymerization begins

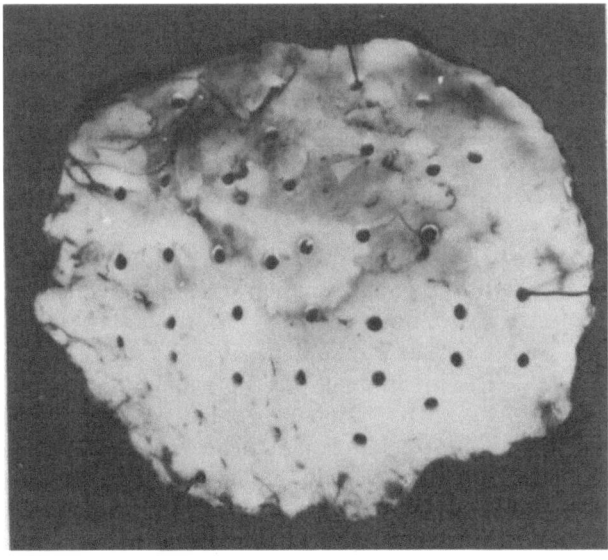

Fig. 65. Polymerized and multiply-perforated Palacos® plastic before incorporation
into the skull defect

irregularities on the upper surface of the prosthesis can be smoothed out with a few drops of monomer (Fig. 64).

When the modelling is finished, the zinc plate is removed together with the bone cement prosthesis. This takes place still in the first phase of the polymerization process (3–5 minutes), where the hardening temperature has not yet increased above 40 °C. The second phase of the polymerization process with tissue-damaging high temperatures does not, therefore, take place in the patient. The necessity of an insulating layer for the dura against heat or the cooling of the prosthesis during the hardening process can be omitted. Moulding the plastic over the zinc plate has also the purpose of giving to the prosthesis an ideal form (Fig. 65).

Small holes, 1–2 cm apart, are drilled in the prosthesis when the hardening process is completed; this should permit any collection of exsudate to drain off or to be removed by tapping. Apart from this, the procedure allows for the growth of connective tissue through the plate, which ultimately results in a better fixation of the latter [61]. The prepared prosthesis is then set into the bone gap and secured on at least two facing sides with mersilene sutures.

"It is superfluous to fix it. The exactness with which it is modelled on to the bone edges ensures a secure fit," wrote Woringer in 1953 in one of his first reports on cranioplasty [184]. Experience has later shown that, in spite of an exact fit, the stability is not guaranteed, especially in the first weeks or months. If a seroma is formed, then the tight sit of an unfixed prosthesis is especially threatened.

In the course of events, several authors [71, 79, 92] secured the transplant with metal loops or Kirschner's wires. Indeed, a perfect stabilization was thereby achieved; however, skin necrosis was not a seldom finding in pressure areas, particularly over a thin or scarred scalp.

Recently, the fixation has been performed with mersilene sutures. A subgaleal redivac drain is inserted for the first 48 hours and the skin closed with deep sitting "Allgöwer" sutures. A subcutaneous suture is not advised because of the danger of suture granuloma and infection. The dressing is changed and the redivac drain removed 48 hours postoperatively. Provided that the wound healing is uneventful, the sutures are removed about 2 weeks after the operation.

This procedure proved to be successful and without complications in the majority of cases. We observed a formation of seroma, which occurred only in cranioplasty performed with bone cements of our patients. The intensity of the seroma depends on the size of the implant; it is usually recognized in the first postoperative week. The treatment is rather simple, we could control this complication in all cases by puncture under aseptic conditions and a compression bandage; the puncture had to be repeated once or twice.

As usual in cases for foreign body implantation, the contact between the implant and patient's own tissue is of importance. In spite of the necrosis, caused by the so-called primary damage (operative damage), the contact between the bone and the plastic is built in the second and third postoperative week by newly formed bone islands which are detectable directly on the cement [32, 110].

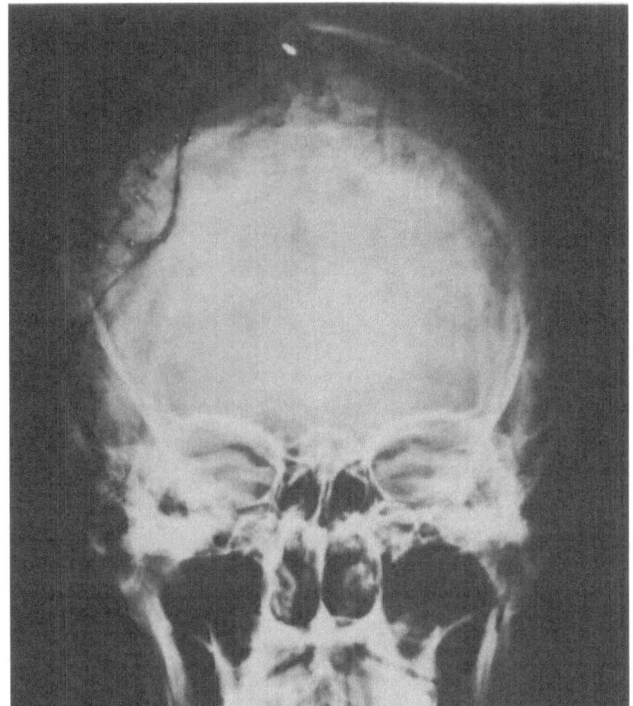

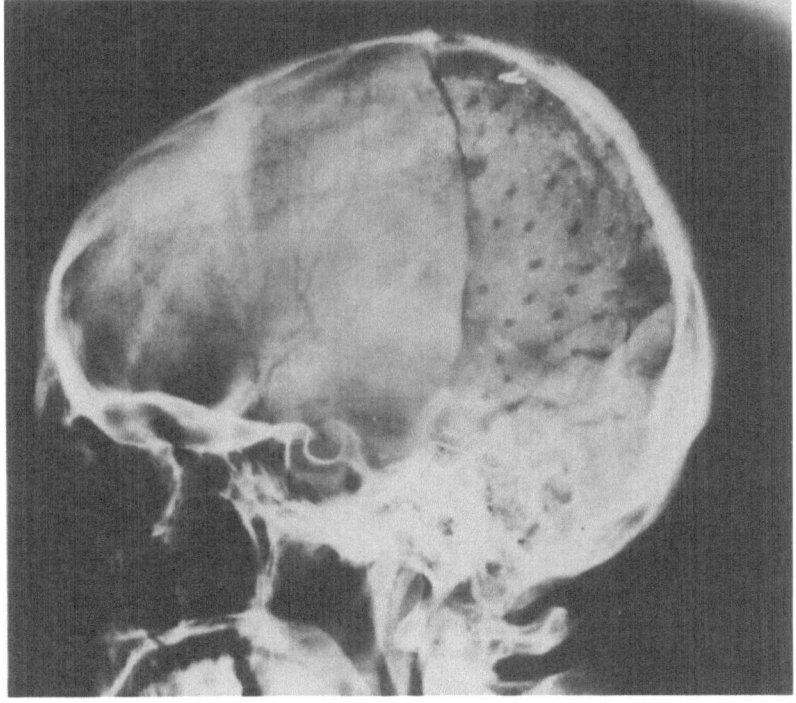

Fig. 66a, b. Cranioplasty with Palacos® R after open craniocerebral injury in parieto-occipital region

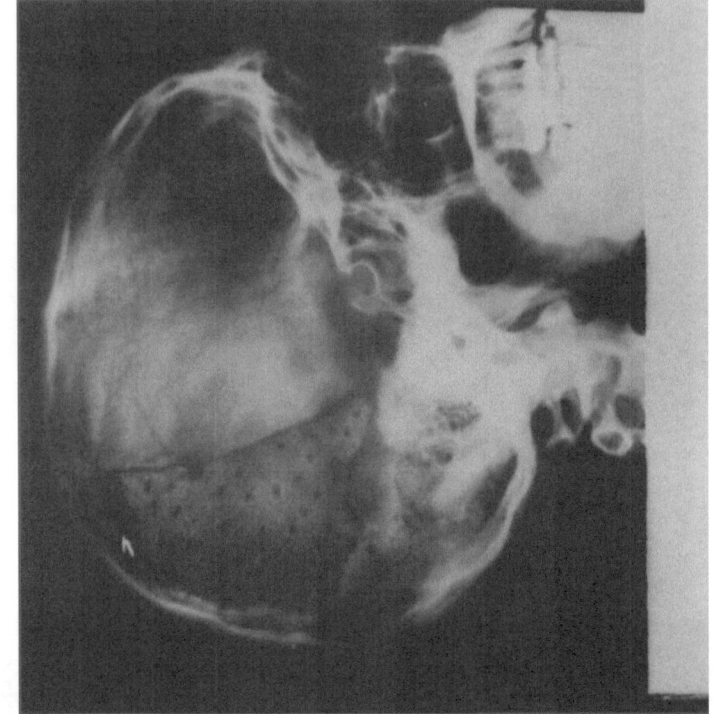

Fig. 67b

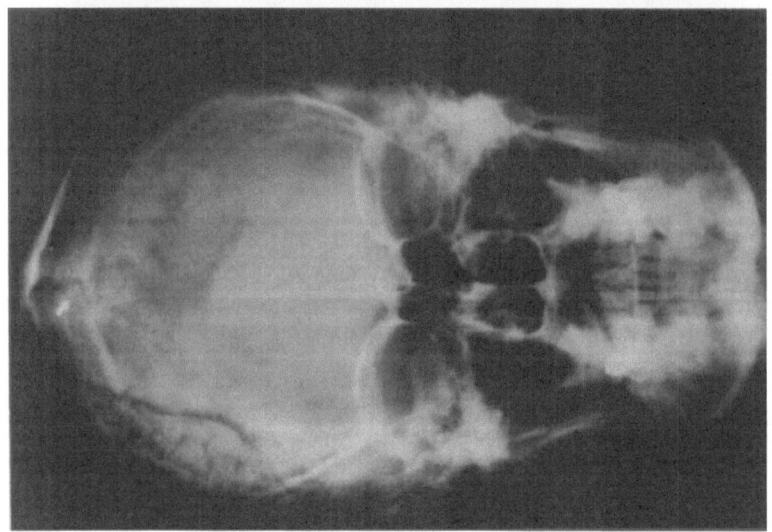

Fig. 67a

Fig. 67a, b. The same patient as in Fig. 66, 10 years later. No detectable changes

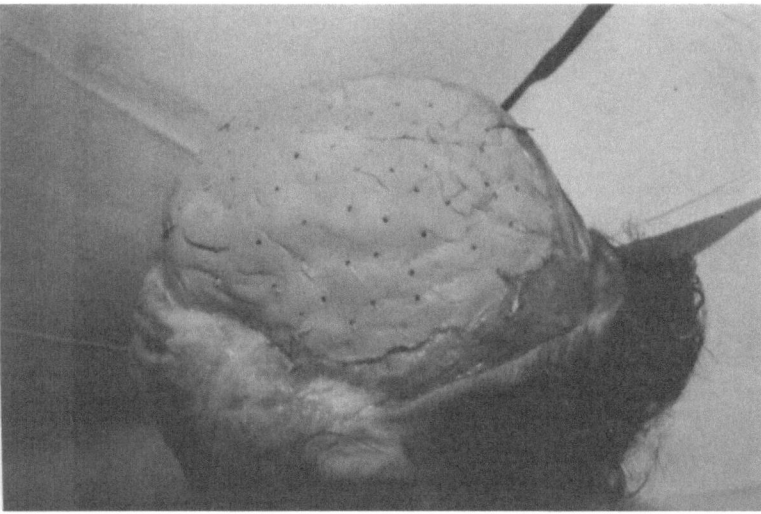

Fig. 68. A 66-year-old patient: She died 4 years after the Palacos® R plastic of a pulmonary embolism. The autopsy shows an irritation-free cranioplasty

Our experience until now with this technique was satisfactory and showed that cranioplasty with bone cements in general not only succeeded in an optimal cosmetic result, but also guaranteed a maximal tissue protection. Exemplary cases are illustrated in Figs. 66 (a, b), 67 (a, b), and 68.

D. Complications of Cranioplasty

I. Complications with Bone Transplants

Of 95 cranial repairs performed with bone grafts, which represents 43,8% of the total plastic operations carried out during a period of ca. 10 years, 11 were carried out with homologous bone. One year later, we found 8 of these bone grafts totally resorbed.

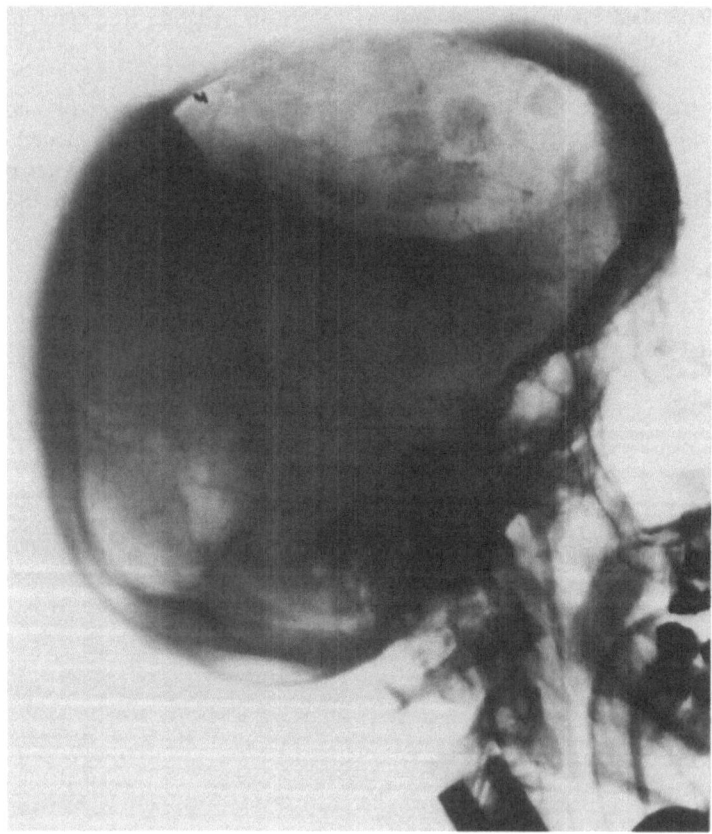

Fig. 69. Practically total resorption of the patient's own bone after cranioplasty 18 months before

Eighty-four of our patients underwent cranioplasty with their own bone, which was in 78 cases conserved in the bone bank. As mentioned before, in the 6 other patients, the cranioplasty was carried out with a bone graft which had been conserved under the abdominal wall of the patient. From 1969 until 1977 we used to perform multiple perforations in the bone graft to allow better drainage of the epidural space. This procedure was used in 57% of cases. We registered practically complete resorption of the bone in more than half (65%) of all such grafts within 12–18 months postoperatively; signs of partial bone resorption were found in 11 patients, and in only 6 patients with perforated bone grafts we did not observe signs of bone resorption within the first year after cranioplasty.

In 36 operated patients (from 1977 until the end of 1980), repaired with non-perforated bone grafts, no signs of bone resorption were found at a check-up 12 months later. Among these patients were also 6 patients with bone grafts which had been conserved under the abdominal wall. We could control only 26 patients two years after surgical repair of the skull. At this time we found 11 completely and 6 partially absorbed bone lids. Such a high percentage of osteolysis of the bone grafts has also been reported by other authors [72, 156].

II. Complications After the Use of Bone Cements

Cranioplasty with Bone cement® or Palacos® R *without* the addition of antibiotics was undertaken in 51 patients during the period from 1969 until the middle of 1975. Since 1975 cranioplasty operations were performed almost exclusively with bone cements to which antibiotics were added (Riphocim-Palacos® R or Palacos® R with Garamycin®).

Altogether 71 cranial repairs were performed with such a material. Cranioplasty performed with Palacos® R or Bone Cement® had to be removed because of infection in ca. 14% of cases. Wound infections in patients with cranioplasty performed with acrylates to which antibiotics were added were observed, by contrast, in 8.5% of cases. It seems, therefore, that there is a relevant difference in the frequency of infection between the patients in whom bone cements with or without the addition of antibiotics were used. This is in agreement with the findings of other authors that [17, 97, 175, 176] the antibiotics are released from the prosthesis into the vicinity of the implant.

Of a total of 122 patients with an acrylate prosthesis, the prosthesis had to be removed in 4 patients within the first 3 months postoperatively because of the necrosis of the scalp. In a few cases with a large prosthesis, we observed a seroma formation in the subgaleal space immediately after the operation. This can be considered as an irritation effect due to a foreign body [174]. We punctured the seromas of all these patients, sometimes removing more than 50 ml of the liquid. Such a puncture, however, is per se connected with the impending danger of an infection. But not recognizing as well as not removing the exudate early enough, leads to infection in most of the cases and finally to the removal of the plastic closure [141].

The danger of later complications in bone cements cranioplasty is considerably reduced if the postoperative course during the first 12–16 weeks is uneventful. We recorded no undesirable effects of any kind later than 6 months after insertion of a methylmethacrylate prosthesis. Taking into account all postoperative troubles, we have had a complication rate of only 14% in cranioplasty performed with bone cements, which is in agreement with findings of other authors [42, 114, 128]. Comparing to a total rate of 70.5% of complications after the use of bony material, there is no doubt that cranial repair with bone cements, preferably combined with antibiotics, is much more advantageous. In Table 9 the frequency of various complications after cranioplasty with different materials is presented.

Table 9. *Complications of Cranioplasty Operations 1969–1980*

	n opera-tions	Infec-tions	Skin-necrosis	Resorption			Compli-cations total (in %)
				partial	complete	total	
Cranioplasty with bone cement:							
– *with* antibiotics: (Riphocim–Palacos® R, Palacos® R with Garamycin R)	71	6					
– *without* antibiotics: (Bone Cement, Palacos® R)	51	7	4	–	–	–	17 (13.9)
total	122	13	4	–	–	–	17 (13.9)
Cranioplasty with bone:							
– autologous:	84						
– perforated	48	–	–	11	31	42	42 (87.5)
– non-perforated	36	–	–	6	11	17	17 (47.2)
– homologous	11	–	–	–	8	8	8 (72.7)
total	95	–	–	17	50	67	67 (70.5)

E. Cranioplasty in Children

I. General

The plastic closure of cranial defects in children confronts the neuro-surgeon with special problems. Large and especially pulsating defects are not well tolerated by children, since the immaturity of the brain can hardly resist the continuous stress of locally changing pressure fluctuations [95, 158]. Moreover, neurological deficits caused by hemisphere compression can strongly influence the further development of the child (Figs. 70a, b).

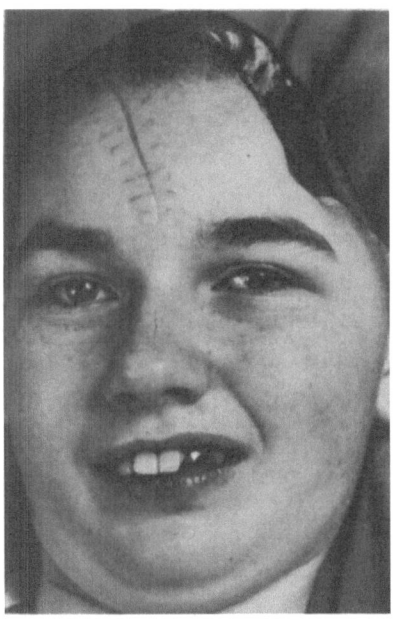

Fig. 70a

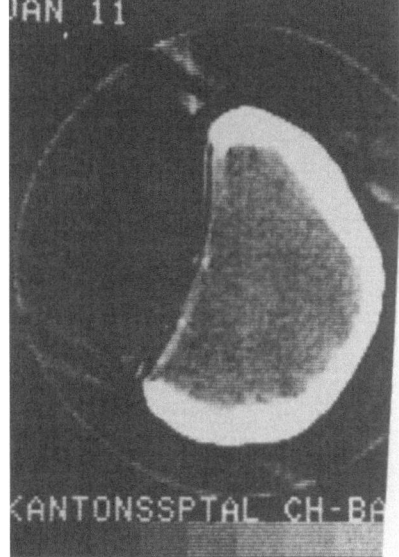

Fig. 70b

Fig. 70a. A 13-year-old girl with a large cranial bone defect after removal of an acute subdural haematoma. Severe psychoorganic syndrome, aphasia with hemiparesis on the right

Fig. 70b. CT of the skull: marked brain mass displacement with collapse and deformation of the hemisphere

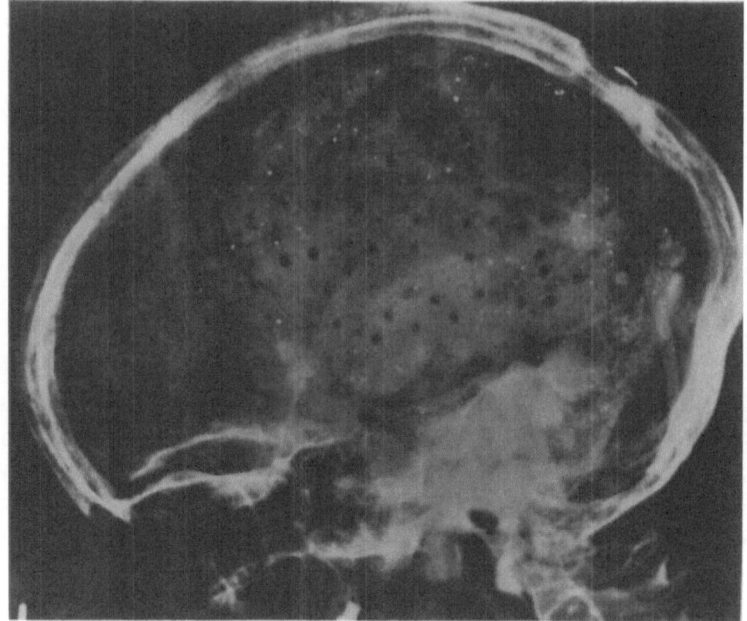

Fig. 71a

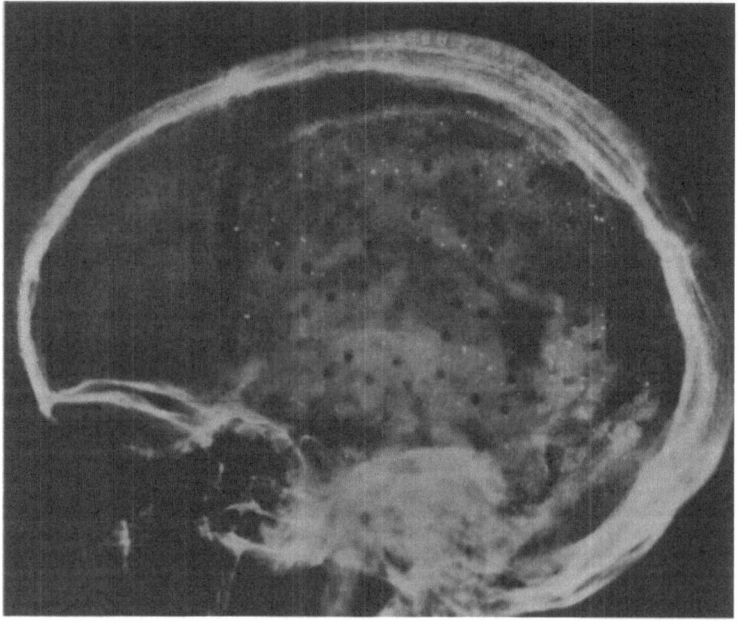

Fig. 71b

Fig. 71a. Cranioplasty with Palacos® R (right parietal) after decompression craniotomy in a 12-year-old girl with acute subdural haematoma

Fig. 71b. The same patient as in Fig. 71a, 5 years later

In the last 11 years (1969–1980) we have performed cranioplasty in only 14 (6.5%) young patients. All children had craniocerebral injuries. The youngest patient was 5 years old and the oldest 13 years old. Five children received their own bone reimplanted, and in the 9 others we used a modified method of Woringer with quick-hardening acrylate (Palacos® R) [160]. Already after the first experiences it was obvious that cranioplasty using perforated own bone shows, as is the case in adults, marked signs of resorption. Two years after operation 11 bone plastics were so strongly affected by resorption changes that they were neither functional nor aesthetic.

By contrast, only one out of nine skull closures performed with acrylates had to be removed due to slackening. In fact, this was a small size defect (2 cm) in the right frontal region caused by an open cranio-cerebral injury. The defect practically completely closed itself with newly formed bone and forced the plastic out. Illustrative is another case of cranioplasty, performed with Palacos® R, in a 12-year-old girl after removal of an acute subdural haematoma. The surface area of the plastic was over 70 cm², but the girl's progress was without complications. No changes of the prosthesis were observed at control examination 5 years later. The cranioplasty still sat perfectly in the 17-year-old normally developed girl. We could detect neither bone defects on the edge of the plastic caused by skull growth nor any other skull deformation (Figs. 71 a, b).

Cranioplasty performed with acrylates in children was not prone to infection. We recorded no such cases.

II. Special Problems of Cranioplasty in Children

The type of plastic operation and the right moment to cover the defect differ in some respects from the procedure in adults. In many cases it is *a priori* not possible to use the child's own bone since it is not available for different reasons (destruction of the bone by tumour infiltration or open craniocerebral injuries). Until recently, most authors advocated against the use of acrylates for cranial repair, because an excessive reaction of the child to the foreign body was feared [95, 114]. Apart from this, it was considered that the child grows out of the inserted bone lid in the course of the development. For this reason, it was generally recommended to close the defect with rib pieces, the wing of the ileum or with a foreign bone [74, 114, 164]. All these procedures require, however, a second operation with a corresponding blood loss. Moreover, the bone is resorbed in more than 75% of the cases [34].

In the last few years, a return to the use of acrylates for the cranioplasty in children could be observed; this was especially favoured by american authors [120, 180, 185].

The healing tendency of infantile skull bones can enormously differ. On the one side, spontaneous bone closure of very large traumatic gaps or trepanations can sometimes occur [19, 55], but on the other side, a stand-still or even an enlargement of the fissure ("growing skull fracture") could be observed. In the later case, the initially narrow and only slightly gaping fracture line is not closed, rather it grows wider, the defect enlarges, whereby metaplastic processes occur on the bone edges, occasionally with new bone formation. Tearing of the dura mater with interposition between the bone edges, cerebrospinal fluid escape with formation of a "meningiocele spurie", and absorption processes on the edges of the fissure, are prerequisites for such condition [19, 55, 95].

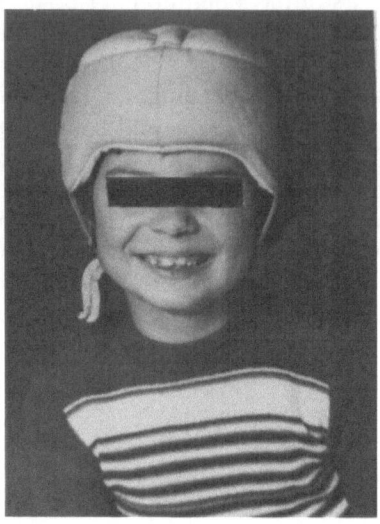

Fig. 72. A 10-year-old child with a protection helmet

Several examples reported by Bushe years ago, showed that a spontaneous regeneration of the cranial bone and spontaneous closure of the defect in young people is possible [19]. Therefore, it is of advantage to wait with a plastic repair, especially in skull defects covered with muscles. When no spontaneous bone formation appears after 1–2 years, a surgical intervention can be taken into consideration. On the other side, when the brain surface in cranial defects is only covered by skin and dura, then an additional brain injury because of the missing brain protection (skull bone) is often feared. In our opinion this fear is exaggerated, since we observed no additional accidents in our young patients [158]. In order to prevent injury, specially made protective helmets could be prescribed by paediatricians. The helmets as worn by our patients are of hard leather. They are tied under the chin and resemble the head protection of a rugby player (Fig. 72). Such helmets, whatever their construction might be, represent, however, a mental and physical burden for children, just to mention the mocking to which they are sometimes exposed, particularly from their classmates and other children.

In general, and as a rule, every defect exceeding 3 cm in diameter should be closed as early as possible [19, 55, 120]. In view of the progress in technical means and surgical methods in the recent years, our experience and that of other authors [120] suggests that it is not advisable to repair a skull defect in a child, where the patient's own bone is missing, with autologous or homoplastic bone material. A cranioplasty with bone cements combined with antibiotics offers considerable advantages, since it can save the child from further surgical interventions and the risks with which they are combined [6]. The perfect aesthetic and clinical success of cranial repair in a child is illustrated in Figs. 73a, b.

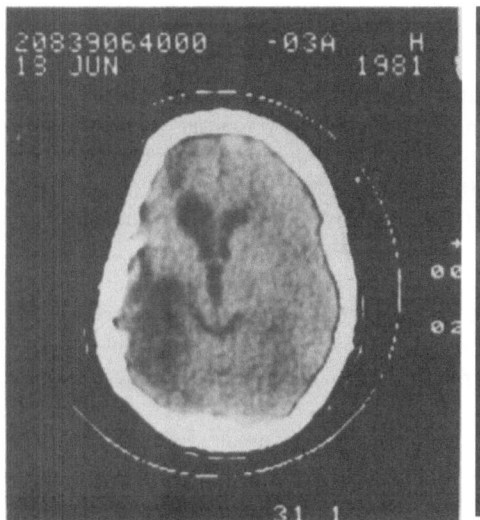 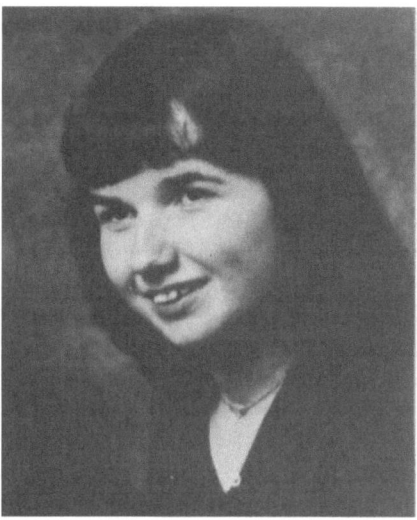

Fig. 73a   Fig. 73b

Fig. 73a. CT of the skull after cranioplasty. Brain mass displacement has regressed, signs of the severe injury 3½ years before are still obvious

Fig. 73b. The same patient as in Fig. 70a, 3½ years later

We recommend even in cases where the paranasal sinuses are open to first try a cranioplasty with antibiotic-containing bone cements in spite of differing opinions [85, 95, 131, 156] which existed before the more recent investigations have shown that antibiotics from the bone cements (Palacos® R with Garamycin®) are released into the vicinity of the prosthesis in a concentration which is considered an effective prophylaxis against infection [17, 133, 176]. The functional and aesthetic results of cranial repair by means of bone cement cannot be surpassed by any other method [132]. In the case that after some years the prosthesis becomes "too small", then it can be replaced in quite a simple manner [158].

F. General Conclusion

Since the beginning of the last century neurosurgeons and traumatologists have been concerned with the question of how to close a primary or secondary skull gap in the most optimal way. The literature, which grew extensively since then, described a great variety of different operating techniques and of the materials used [36, 149]. The diversity of the procedures demonstrated that there was no general agreement about the method of choice.

After World War II, due to continuous increase in the frequency of severe craniocerebral injuries, the problem of skull defect closure received even more attention. Protective and cosmetic aspects of cranial repair lost their primary importance: new indications were recognized, and by consequence new operating techniques were developed [183].

To deal with intracranial processes means to deal with exceptional problems. No other cavity of the body is surrounded with such rigid walls as the cranium, which is, in addition, divided into several subcompartments by sheets of dura. Nowhere else in the body, therefore, are displacements of the contents by space occupying processes as complicated in their dynamics as in the inner cavity of the skull and, not to forget, taking place in such functionally highly differentiated organ. Brain functions, vascularization of vessels and CSF flow are often considerably impaired by the appearance of pathological intracranial processes, sometimes even in a life-threatening manner [124, 139].

Intracranial changes which develop in uncovered defects were not sufficiently known in the past. This problem has gained a new dimension after the introduction of computerized tomography. It is noteworthy that the first documented observations of clinical deterioration which was related to the presence of large cranial defect was published only in 1976.

Tabaddor and La Morgese described their case as follows [162]:

"Four months after removal of a subarachnoid haematoma with decompressive craniotomy, a 41 year old patient showed a left progressive hemisyndrome which was directly proportional to the concavity of the skin flap over the skull defect."

The pathogenesis of the progressive neurological symptoms which appeared 120 days after the operation was at that time not clear. The carotisangiogram showed a midline displacement, and the "dynamic scintigram" revealed a reduced circulation on the side of the operation. After the closure of the defect the authors observed the regression of the neurological deficit within a few days, one month later a symmetrical flow of both hemispheres was restored and the patient was able to return to normal daily life.

Since the deteriorations and improvements were not analyzed by computer tomography, the deeply pitted skin flap, supposed to be responsible for the formation of these complications, was explained by the difference between atmospheric and intracranial pressure.

One year later the japanese authors Yamara and Makino [186] reported their experience in 33 patients with cranial defects. In some patients intracranial changes were examined by computer tomography for the first time. Neurological symptoms appearing in the postoperative course or deteriorations of already existing neurological deficiencies, found in nearly 30% of the cases, were attributed to brain mass displacement, hemisphere deformation and ventricle collapse.

Also, these authors postulated the difference between intracranial and atmospheric pressure as reason for this condition and indicated that patients with pitted or flat skin flaps and neurological deficiencies of a moderate degree (slight aphasia, mono- or hemiparesis without a marked disability, psycho-organic syndrome with retained orientation) have the best chance for a post-operative improvement and a neurological restitution.

These findings are largely in accordance with our observations. Of 22 (20.7%) patients with neurological deficiencies, except for one patient, none completely improved postoperatively. Partial recovery was observed in 9% of patients. All these patients have had sunken-in skin flaps.

By contrast, patients with less pronounced neurological symptoms, irrespectively of the size of the defect and with flat or normal skin flaps, proved to have the best prognosis and the best chances of recovery. Almost the half (48%) of these patients showed complete regression of the neurological deficiencies in the postoperative period after the closure of the defect. In further 35% of the cases we have observed partial recovery. Nearly two thirds of these patients had sunken-in skin flaps.

Decisive role for the postoperative recovery of patients with cranial defects play, therefore, the severity of the symptoms, the size of the bone defect and the condition of the skin flap. There is no doubt today that neurological and psychic symptoms which appear in the course of time in large cranial defects, or deterioration of already existing neurological deficiencies, are due to intra-cranial changes [158, 162, 167, 186].

The examinations by means of computer tomography have indicated that the normalization of the intracranial situation after cranioplasty is in all probability the main reason for the rapid improvement of the symptomatology. Since its introduction practically all our patients have been examined by computer tomography before and after cranioplasty. In most cases, already within a few days after the closure of the skull defect, a normalization of the intracranial situation, i.e. regression of brain mass displacement, expansion of the brain and normalization of the ventricles was demonstrated. There were a few cases where the return to the normal position of the intracranial contents was not achieved, especially there where the process existed over a longer period of time and where adhesions between dura and brain surface were present. Moreover, atrioventricular shunts, inserted because of internal posttraumatic hydrocephalus, were also the cause of the normalization failure.

Of 20 patients with epileptic fits examined electroencephalographically, 11 (55%) showed an improvement in the postoperative course: hard waves and spikes as well as the focal disturbances disappeared. A general stabilization of the EEG was observed. In spite of this, the influence of cranioplasty on epilepsy, is not yet a resolved question [43]. We assume that cranial repair has a positive effect on epileptic disorders, but more extensive investigations are necessary in order to prove this. The fact is that more than a half of our patients showed clinical as well as EEG signs of the decreased convulsion potential accompanied by a normalization of the intracranial situation. It should be mentioned, however, that it was recently reported that in about one third of the patients with posttraumatic epilepsy, the seizures stopped spontaneously within 2 years, regardless of whether cranioplasty was performed or not [177]. According to these observation the time of performing cranioplasty is, therefore, irrelevant.

In our view, however, the time chosen for surgery does play a role because most posttraumatic forms of epilepsy develop 3–6 months after the injury. Therefore, the effect of the "Sinking Skin Flap Syndrome" (pitted wound with brain mass displacement and ventricle deformation) which is often found in large skull defects, must be regarded as an important cause or at least a facilitating factor in its development. It is possible that cranial repair represents only one component in the therapy of postoperative epilepsy. Adequate controlled treatment with anticonvulsants is undoubtedly the second important approach in the treatment of these posttraumatic complications [151].

Scintigraphic examinations which were carried out in 10 of our patients, showed clear-cut circulatory disturbances in the region of the uncovered hemisphere. After cranioplasty symmetrical circulation was restored.

Since computerized tomography examinations in patients with sinking skin-flap syndrome have detected changes similar to those of intracranial space occupying processes with raised intracranial pressure, intracranial pressure monitoring in these patients was warranted in order to objectively clarify this problem. We supposed that similar clinical pathology in both patient groups (intracranial space occupying processes or large cranial bone defects) may have similar patho-anatomical cause. Continuous pre- and postoperative epidural pressure monitoring indeed identified raised intracranial pressure in 58% of such patients. A normalization of the pressure was observed in these patients shortly after the repair of the skull defect. In some, however, in whom the intracranial pressure was within the normal limits before and after cranioplasty, intracranial changes which could be characterized as "mild" were found; the clinical symptomatology was also not impressive. At present it cannot be explained why practically no pathological changes were found in these few patients in spite of the large skull defects. Perhaps, this could be ascribed to exceptional adaption ability of the brain, as sometimes observed in patients with only slowly growing intracranial processes.

The main problem in the plastic repair of skull defects is the choice of material.

In our own experience cranioplasty with bones was not satisfactory. Reports of several authors [9] that a bony consolidation of the graft using conserved foreign bone occurred in more than half of the patients could not be confirmed by our results. Over 72% of all our bone lids were resorbed after about a year. Likewise, the results when using the patient's own bone, which had been stored in the bone bank at a temperature of $-25\,°C$, were disappointing. In a period of 1–2 years partial or complete resorption of the prosthesis was found in over 70% of the cases. The best and the most successful proved to be the use of bone cements: in only 13.9% complications (infections, skin necrosis) occurred. The frequency of unwanted effects is even less if bone cements with antibiotics are used.

There is no general agreement about the optimal time for performing a repair of cranial defect. We are of the opinion that in the case of local infection (for instance after previous cranioplasty or because of other reasons) a defect closure – regardless of the material used – should be carried out at the earliest after 10–12 months. Even in exceptional cases, for example in patients with increasing neurological dysfunctions or with deeply pitted wounds or threatening brain mass displacement, cranioplasty should be performed at the earliest 3 months after the infection has been completely cured.

The value of cranioplasty is primarily in its prophylactic but in many cases also therapeutic effect. Based on these facts, two important indications for cranioplasty can be deduced: prevention or correction of already existing intracranial changes in large unprotected cranial defects. Due to the present state of the art, there are almost no contraindications for cranioplasty. Even if the paranasal sinuses are open and communicating with the brain cavity, no major problems are encountered if bone cements combined with antibiotics and appropriate surgical technique are used. The simple application, very good tissue tolerance, cosmetic success and, last but not least, the reasonable cost of the operation [15] recommend cranioplasty with bone cements as the method of choice.

In conclusion, cranioplasty has today undoubtedly an important place in the reconstructive surgery because of the following reasons:

- restoration of the displaced bone and tissue mass, together with normalization of the intracranial conditions,
- positive effect on epileptic seizures in some patients,
- normalization of the retarded cerebral circulation on the uncovered side of the brain, and
- normalization of the intracranial pressure in the majority of patients after closure of the cranial defect.

Last but not least, its psychological and cosmetic effects should not be neglected.

References

1. Aust, W.: Beitrag zur Transplantation mit alloplastischem Material bei Knochendefekten des Schädels. Chirurg *23/1*, 19–22 (1952).
2. Ahyai, A., Schmitt, E.: Late Intracranial Infection after Tantalum Cranioplasty. Neurochirurgia *25*, 103–104 (1982).
3. Axhausen, G.: Zur Technik der Schädelplastik. Langenbecks Arch. klin. Chir. *107*, 551–574 (1916).
4. Baltensweiler, J., Clodius, L., Eberle, H.: Autologe Schädeldachplastik. Helv. chir. Acta *43*, 717–719 (1976).
5. Bart, A.: Über künstliche Erneuerung von Knochengewebe über die Ziele der Osteoplastik. Berl. Klin. Wschr. *33*, 8–11 (1896).
6. Bauer, M., Hussl, H., Anderl, H., Wilflingseder, P.: Grundsätze, Methoden und Resultate der Versorgung von Stirnbeindefekten. Chirurg *45*, 514–518 (1974).
7. Belopavlovic, M., Buchthal, A., Beks, J. W. F., Journée, H. L.: Some Principles of Postoperative Epidural Pressure Monitoring. Acta Neurochir. (Wien) *55*, 227–245 (1981).
8. Berndt, F.: Über den Verschluß von Schädeldefekten durch Periost-Knochenlappen von der Tibia. Dtsch. Z. Chir. *48*, 620–623 (1898).
9. Bettag, W.: Über homoioplastische Deckungen von Schädellücken. Acta Neurochir. (Wien) Suppl. III, 36–40 (1955).
10. Bier, A., Braun, H., Kümmel, H.: Chirurgische Operationslehre, 8. Aufl., Bd. 2/I, pp. 71–75. Leipzig: J. A. Barth. 1973.
11. Black, S. P. W., Kam, C. C. M., Sights, W. P., Jr.: Aluminium Cranioplasty. J. Neurosurg. *29*, 562–564 (1968).
12. Boswick, J.: The Use of Betadine-Antiseptics in Treating Burns and Other Wounds at the Hand. In: Proceedings at the World Congress on Antisepsis, VI. 1970, HP Publishing Co., Inc., New York. 1970.
13. Braley, S. A.: The Use of Silicones in Plastic Surgery. A Retrospective View. Plast. Reconstr. Surg. *51*, 280–288 (1973).
14. Breuel, H. P., Emrich, D.: Untersuchung der zerebralen Durchblutung. In: Nuklearmedizinische Funktionsdiagnostik und Therapie (Emrich, D., ed.), p. 244. Stuttgart: G. Thieme Verlag. 1979.
15. Bricolo, A., Benati, A., Bazzan, A.: Cranioplastiche con resina acrilica, con rete di acciaio inossidabile pesante e con frammenti di teca. Minerva Neurochirurgica *11*, 208–211 (1967).
16. Brown, K. E.: Fabrication of an Alloplastic Cranioimplant. J. Pros. Dent. *8*, 213–224 (1970).
17. Buchholz, H. W., Engelbrecht, H.: Über die Depotwirkung einiger Antibiotica bei Vermischung mit dem Kunstharz Palacos. Chirurg *40/11*, 511–515 (1970).
18. Busch, J.: Die Trepanation seit Beginn der modernen Chirurgie. Ciba Zeitschr. Nr. 39, 1936.

19. Bushe, K. A.: Spontane Regeneration traumatischer und operativer Knochendefekte des Schädels. Zbl. Neurochir. *21/6*, 337–348 (1961).

20. Cabanela, M. E., Coventry, M. B., Maccarty, C. S., Miller, W. E.: The Fate of Patients with Methyl Methacrylate Cranioplasty. J. Bone Jt. Surg. *54-A/2*, 278–281 (1972).

21. Cain, H., Carstensen, G.: Morphologische Grundlagen für die Verwendung einer neuartigen „Gefäßbank" im Tierexperiment. Langenbecks Arch. klin. Chir. *296*, 88–101 (1960).

22. Campell, E., Meirosky, A., Pompkins, V.: Studies on the Use of Metals in Surgery (Part II). Ann. Surg. *116*, 763–775 (1942).

23. Chapiro, H. M., Wyte, S. R., Loeser, J.: Barbiturate-augmented Hypothermia for Reduction of Persistent Intracranial Hypertension. J. Neurosurg. *40*, 90–100 (1974).

24. Charitonowa, K. K.: Ersatz von Schädeldefekten durch Hornplatten. Fragen der Neurochir. *4*, 37 (1952) (Russ.).

25. Clodius, L.: Knorpeltransplantationen in der plastischen Chirurgie. Bull. schweiz. Akad. med. Wiss. *18*, 277–286 (1970).

26. Conley, J.: Use of Composite Flaps Containing Bone for Major Repairs in the Head and Neck. Plast. Reconstr. Surg. *49/5*, 522–526 (1972).

27. Crout, D. H. G., Corkill, J. A., James, M. L., Ling, R. S. M.: Methylmethacrylate Metabolism in Man. Clin. Orthop. *141*, 90–95 (1979).

28. Debrunner, H. U.: Die Erwärmung von Knochenzement bei Polymerisation. Arch. orthop. Unfall-Chir. *78*, 309–318 (1974).

29. Diener, A., Dörr, N., Herrmann, K. O.: Untersuchungen und Ergebnisse der physikalischen und physiologischen Gesetzmäßigkeiten bei der Anwendung von Kunststoff in der Knochenchirurgie. Zbl. Chir. *46*, 2376–2381 (1956).

30. Dietz, H.: Die frontobasale Schädelhirnverletzung, pp. 6–7. Berlin-Heidelberg-New York: Springer. 1970.

31. Dietz, H., Umbach, W., Wüllenweber, R.: Klinische Neurochirurgie, Band I, pp. 79–85. Stuttgart-New York: G. Thieme Verlag. 1982.

32. Draenert, K., Rudigier, J., Herrmann, W., Willenegger, H.: Tierexperimentelle Studie zur Histomorphologie des Knochen-Zement-Kontaktes. Helv. chir. Acta *43*, 769–773 (1976).

33. Drevermann, P.: Über den Ersatz von Dura und Schädeldefekten, unter besonderer Berücksichtigung der Dauererfolge in der Verhütung und Heilung der traumatisierten Epilepsie durch Duraersatz mit frei transplantiertem Fettgewebe. Bruns Beitr. Klin. Chir. *127*, 674–697 (1922).

34. Eberle, H.: Das Schicksal tiefgefrorener autoplastischer Schädelkalottenreimplantate nach Schädel-Hirn-Trauma. Helv. chir. Acta *43*, 713–716 (1976).

35. Ecke-Giessen, H.: Neue Wege der quantitativen Bestimmung der ossären Regeneration an Knochentransplantaten. Langenbecks Arch. Chir. *319*, 448–450 (1967).

36. Ehmer, D., Krumbholz, S., Kaufmann, E.: Zur Problematik der Deckung von Schädelkalottendefekten mit Methakrylaten. Zbl. Chir. *31*, 1054–1059 (1971).

37. Ehrlich, I., Kricun, M. E., Gonzalez, C. F.: EMI Scan Density of Methyl Methacrylate. Amer. J. Roentgenol. *129*, 351–352 (1977).

38. v. Eiselberg, A.: Zur Behandlung von erworbenen Schädelknochendefekten. Zbl. Chir. *22*, Beil. Nr. 27, 44 (1895).

39. Ekstedt, J.: CSF Hydrodynamic Studies in Man. Method of Constant Pressure CSF Infusion. J. Neurol. Neurosurg. Psychiatry *40*, 105–119 (1977).

40. Ekstedt, J.: CSF Hydrodynamic Studies in Man. Normal Hydrodynamic Variables Related to CSF Pressure and Flow. J. Neurol. Neurosurg. Psychiatry *41*, 345–353 (1978).

41. Elkins, Ch. W., Cameron, J. E.: Cranioplasty with Acrylic Plates. J. Neurosurg. *3*, 199–205 (1946).

42. Elkins, Ch. W., Holbrook, T.: In: Late Complications Following Cranioplasty with Alloplastic Plates (White, I. C., ed.). Ann. Surg. *128*, 743–755 (1948).

43. Erculei, F., Walker, A. E.: Posttraumatic Epilepsy and Early Cranioplasty. J. Neurosurg. *20/12*, 1085–1089 (1963).

44. Faulhauer, K., Fischer, D.: Erfahrungen mit der Deckung von Schädeldefekten durch Reimplantation gefrierkonservierter Knochenlappen und durch Tantalplastiken. Chir. plastica *1*, 361–373 (1973).

45. Finseth, F., Cutting, C.: An Experimental Neurovascular Island Skin Flap for the Study of the Delay Phenomenon. Plast. Reconstr. Surg. *61/3*, 412–420 (1978).

46. Flörcken, H.: Großer traumatischer Defekt des Stirnschädels. Ersatz durch eine Plexiglasplatte. Chirurg *27/4*, 178–180 (1956).

47. Fodstad, H., Ekstedt, J.: Liquordynamik bei ausgedehnten Knochendefekten. Vortrag anl. des Kongr. „Union Schweiz. Chir. Fachges." in Basel, 8.–10. Juni, 1977. Schweiz. Arch. Neurol. Neurochir. Psych. *123/2*, 225 (1978).

48. Fraenkel, A.: Überdeckung von Trepanationsdefekten am Schädel durch Heteroplastik. Wien. klin. Wochenschr. *3*, 475–476 (1890).

49. Fulcher, O. H.: Tantalum as a Metallic Implant to Repair Cranial Defects. J.A.M.A. *121/12*, 931–933 (1943).

50. Gaab, M., Knoblich, O. E., Dietrich, K.: Miniaturisierte Methoden zur Überwachung des intrakraniellen Druckes. Langenbecks Arch. Chir. *350*, 13–31 (1979).

51. Gänshirt, H.: Der Hirnkreislauf, pp. 350–375, 719–728. Stuttgart: G. Thieme Verlag. 1972.

52. Galicich, J. H., Hovind, K. H.: Stainless Steel Mesh-Acrylic Cranioplasty. J. Neurosurg. *27*, 376–378 (1967).

53. Gardner, W. J.: Tantal in the Immediate Repair of Traumatic Skull Defects. Method of Immobilizing the Wounded Brain. Nav. med. Bull. Wash. *43*, 1100–1106 (1944).

54. Gardner, W. J.: Closure of Defect of the Skull with Tantalum. Surg. Gynec. Obstet. *80*, 303–312 (1975).

55. Gerlach, J., Jensen, H. P., Koos, W., Kraus, H.: Pädiatrische Neurochirurgie, pp. 218–223, 463. Stuttgart: G. Thieme Verlag. 1967.

56. Gerlach, J.: Grundriß der Neurochirurgie, pp. 108–111. Darmstadt: Dr. Dietrich Steinkopf Verlag. 1967.

57. Gerlitt, J.: Der Trepan. Ciba Zeitschr. 39, 1936.

58. Gobiet, W.: Ergebnisse intrakranieller Druckmessungen im akuten post-traumatischen Stadium. Anaesthesist *26*, 187–195 (1977).

59. Gobiet, W., Bock, W., Liesegang, J., Grotze, W.: Experience with an intracranial pressure transducer readjustable in vivo. J. Neurosurg. *40*, 272–276 (1976).

60. Gobiet, W.: Intensivtherapie nach Schädel-Hirn-Trauma. Berlin-Heidelberg-New York: Springer. 1977.

61. Göhring, K.: Beitrag zur alloplastischen Deckung von Schädeldefekten mit einem autopolymerisierenden Kunststoff. Med. Klin. *23*, 1020–1023 (1960).

62. Goldhaber, P.: Preliminary Observations on Bone Isografts within Diffusion Chambers. Proc. Soc. Exptl. Biol. Med. *98*, 53–56 (1958).

63. Glowacki, J., Murray, J. E., Kaban, L. B., Folkman, J., Mulliken, J. B.: Application of the Biological Principle of Induced Osteogenesis for Craniofacial Defects. The Lancet, May 2, 1981.

64. Gottlob, R., Blümel, G.: Verwendung von Klebestoffen – Anastomosierung kleiner Blutgefäße. Aktuelle Chirurgie 5, 287–292 (1966).

65. Grant, F. C., Nacross, N. C.: Repair of Cranial Defects by Cranioplasty. Ann. Surg. 110, 488–512 (1939).

66. Grantham, E. G., Landis, H. P.: Cranioplasty and the Posttraumatic Syndrome. J. Neurosurg. 5, 19–22 (1948).

67. Günther, H.: Zur Indikation der Deckung von Stirndefekten mit autoplastischem Knochen, Knorpel und alloplastischem Material. Fortschritte der Kiefer- und Gesichtschirurgie XII, 247–258 (1967).

68. Guido, L. J., Patterson, R. H., Jr.: Focal Neurological Deficits. Secondary to Intraoperative CSF Drainage: Successful Resolution with an Epidural Blood Patch. J. Neurosurg. 45, 348–351 (1976).

69. Gurdjean, E. S.: Management of Depressed Fractures of the Skull and Old Skull Defects. Ann. Surg. 102, 89–101 (1935).

70. Häuptli, J., Segantini, P.: Neue Aufbewahrungsarten von Schädelkalottenstücken nach dekompressiver Kraniotomie. Helv. chir. Acta 47, 121–124 (1980).

71. Hammon, W. M., Kempe, L. G.: Methylmethacrylate Cranioplasty. Acta Neurochir. (Wien) 25, 69–77 (1971).

72. Hancock, D.: The Fate of Replaced Bone Flaps. J. Neurosurg. 20, 983–984 (1963).

73. Hardt, N., Ammann, J., Wolfensberger, C.: Schädeldachersatzplastik nach traumatischen Defekten. Chir. Praxis 21, 25–32 (1976).

74. Hardt, N., Ammann, J.: Erfahrungen mit 73 Schädeldachersatzplastiken. Helv. chir. Acta 43, 721–723 (1976).

75. Hase, U.: Intrakranielle Druckmessung. Neurochirurgia 21, 84–90 (1978).

76. Hecker, A., Stula, D., Scollo-Lavizzari, G.: EEG-Veränderungen vor und nach Schädeldachplastik. S. A. für Neurol., Neurochir. und Psych. 2, 223 (1981).

77. Henkel, G.: Über die Höhe der Restmonomerabgabe bei verschiedenen Kunststoffen. Deutsche Zahn-, Mund- und Kieferheilkunde 9/10, 377–384 (1961).

78. Henry, H. M., Guerrero, C., Moody, R. A.: Cerebrospinal Fluid Fistula from Fractured Acrylic Cranioplasty Plate. J. Neurosurg. 45, 227–228 (1976).

79. Heppner, F.: Schädeldachplastik mit Kunststoff. Pädiat. Prax. 3, 279–282 (1964).

80. Homsy, Ch. A., Tullos, H. S., Anderson, M. S., Diferrante, N. M., King, J. W.: Some Physiological Aspects of Prosthesis Stabilization with Acrylic Polymer. Clin. Orthop. 83, 317–328 (1972).

81. Hoppe, W.: Tierexperimentelle Untersuchungen über Gewebsreaktionen auf Injektionen von autopolymerisierendem Kunststoff. DZZ. Zahnärztliche Zs. 15, 837–847 (1956).

82. Hupfauer, W., Ulatowski, L.: Die Temperaturentwicklung verschiedener Knochenzemente während des Abhärtungsvorganges. Arch. orthop. Unfall-Chir. 72, 174–184 (1972).

83. Idelberger, G.: Palavit in der operativen Orthopädie. Verh. Dtsch. Orthop. Ges. 42, 354–357 (1955).

84. Idelberger, G.: Knochenkonservierung in Palavit und durch Gefriertrocknung. Verh. Dtsch. Orthop. Ges. 43, 69–71 (1956).

85. Issel, P.: Zur Deckung von Knochendefekten des Schädels mit Plexiglas. Zbl. Neurochir. 2/3, 126–132 (1950).

86. Jackson, E., Back, J. B.: Technique of Methylmethacrylate Cranioplasty Utilizing the Pneumatic Craniotomy. Military Medicine *12*, 1519–1521 (1969).

87. Jahnke, K.: Zur Rekonstruktion der Frontobasis mit Keramikwerkstoffen. Laryng. Rhinol. *59*, 111–115 (1980).

88. Jensen, F., Petersen, N. C.: Repair of Denuded Cranial Bone by Bone Splitting and Free-skin Grafting. J. Neurosurg. *44*, 728–731 (1976).

89. Jentzsch, R.: Kunststoffe in der Wiederherstellungs-Chirurgie des Schädels. Langenbecks Arch. klin. Chir. *291*, 303–309 (1959).

90. Kahn, E., Crosby, E. C., Schneider, R. C., Taren, J. A.: Cranioplasty. Correlative Neurosurgery, Second Edition, pp. 583–586. Springfield, Ill.: Ch. C Thomas Publisher. 1969.

91. Kappis, A.: Zur Deckung von Schädeldefekten. Zbl. Chir. *51*, 897–898 (1915).

92. Keil, W.: Zur Frage der alloplastischen Deckung großer Schädeldefekte mit Kunststoff (Palacos R). Med. Bild *3*, 90–91 (1961).

93. Kleinschmidt, O.: Plexiglas zur Deckung von Schädellücken. Der Chirurg *9*, 273–277 (1941).

94. Kleinschmidt, O.: Die Deckung von Schädelknochenlücken. Operative Chirurgie, pp. 573–579. Berlin-Göttingen-Heidelberg: Springer. 1948.

95. Kloos, K.: Probleme der Schädeldachplastik bei Kindern. Pädiat. Prax. *3*, 443–447 (1964).

96. Klingler, M.: Das Schädelhirntrauma, pp. 84–87. Stuttgart: G. Thieme Verlag. 1968.

97. Knöringer, P.: Sofortdeckung von Schädellücken bei offenen und geschlossenen Impressionsfrakturen des Hirnschädels mit Acrylharzkunststoff. Neurochirurgia *22*, 18–23 (1979).

98. Köhnlein, H. E.: Das mechanische Moment, die Anwendung von Leim zur Transplantatfixierung. Hefte zur Unfallheilkunde *80*, 86–88 (1965).

99. König, F.: Der knöcherne Ersatz großer Schädeldefekte. Zbl. Chir. Leipzig *17*, 497–501 (1890).

100. Körlof, B., Nylén, B., Rietz, K. A.: Bone Grafting of Skull Defects. Plast. Reconstr. Surg. *4*, 378–383 (1973).

101. Kollar, W. A. F., Fueger, G. E.: Szintigraphische Befunde nach Polyacryl-Kranioplastiken. Schweiz. Arch. Neurol. Neurochir. Psychiatrie *1*, 21–25 (1971).

102. Kothe, W., Lang, G.: Die Schädeldachplastik mit schnellhärtenden Acrylaten. Zbl. Chir. *14*, 497–501 (1967).

103. Kreider, G. N.: Repair of Cranial Defect by New Method. J.A.M.A. April *10*, 1024 (1920).

104. Kretschmer, H.: Neurotraumatologie, 1/2, pp. 100–101, 111–112. Stuttgart: G. Thieme Verlag. 1978.

105. Krüger, D. W.: Die plastische Deckung von Schädeldefekten. Zbl. Neurochir. *4/5*, 260–272 (1954).

106. Krüger, G., Haubitz, I., Weinhardt, F., Hoyer, S.: Vergleich von Psychopathologie mit Hirndurchblutung und Hirnstoffwechsel im Verlauf zerebrovaskulärer Insuffizienzen. Fortschr. Med. *8*, 295–338 (1982).

107. Krumbholz, S., Berge, G., Willenberg, E., Barthel, G.: Wertigkeit möglicher Schädeldachersatzplastiken. Zbl. Neurochir. *38*, 281–290 (1977).

108. Kuner, E. H., Weyand, F., Domres, B.: Zur Leistungsfähigkeit autologer Spongiosa bei der Behandlung knöcherner Defekte. Mschr. Unfallheilk. *75*, 189–202 (1972).

109. Kunz, Z.: Neurochirurgie, pp. 11–14. Praha: Státní Zdravotnicke Nakladatelství. 1968.

110. Kunzl, L.: Gewebeverträglichkeit der Polymere Polyäthylen, Polyester und Polyacetalharze. Helv. chir. Acta *43*, 775–777 (1976).

111. Lauber, H. J.: Die plastische Deckung knöcherner Schädeldefekte. Zbl. Chir. *4*, 419–423 (1947).

112. LaLonde, A. A., Gardner, W. J.: Chronic Subdural Hematoma. The New Engl. J. Med. *14*, 493–496 (1948).

113. Lehnartz, E.: Chemische Physiologie. Berlin-Göttingen-Heidelberg: Springer. 1959.

114. Leivy, D. M., Tovi, D.: Autogenous Bone Cranioplasty. Neurochirurgia *13*, 3, 82–86 (1970).

115. Linder, L.: Tissue Reaction to Methyl Methacrylate Monomer. Acta Orthop. Scand. *47*, 3–10 (1976).

116. Markwalder, T. M.: Chronic Subdural Hematomas: a Review. J. Neurosurg. *54*, 637–645 (1981).

117. Marschner, G.: Über den plastischen Verschluß von Schädeldachlücken. Zbl. Chir. *52*, 2121–2127 (1957).

118. Merrem, G.: Die Versorgung der Trepanationslücke mit Fremdknochen. Acta Neurochir. (Wien), Suppl. 3, 31–35 (1955).

119. Meschig, R., Schadewaldt, H.: Schädeltrepanationen in Ostafrika. Hexagon „Roche" *3*, 17–24 (1981).

120. Milhorat, T. H.: Cranioplasty, pp. 75–77. Philadelphia: F. A. Davis Company. 1978.

121. Möller, E., Kopp, H.: Wundkleber in der inneren Medizin. Münch. Med. Wschr. *6*, 346–348 (1968).

122. Myers, M. B., Cherry, G.: Mechanism of the Delay Phenomenon. Plast. Reconstr. Surg. *1*, 52–57 (1969).

123. Nau, H. E.: EEG-Veränderungen bei Schädelhirntumoren, Knochendefekten und Schädeldachplastiken. Neurochir. *6*, 192–195 (1981).

124. Olivecrona, H., Tönnis, W.: Handbuch der Neurochirurgie, Bd. I, pp. 132–137, 143–145, 212–214. Berlin-Göttingen-Heidelberg: Springer. 1959.

125. Olivecrona, H., Tönnis, W.: Handbuch der Neurochirurgie, Bd. III, pp. 47–48. Berlin-Göttingen-Heidelberg: Springer. 1956.

126. Papo, I., Caruselli, G., Luongo, A.: CSF Withdrawal for the Treatment of Intracranial Hypertension in Acute Head Injuries. Acta Neurochir. (Wien) *56*, 191–199 (1981).

127. Pavlova, M. N., Vyalcev, V. V.: Autoplasty and Homoplasty of Extensive Defects of the Vault. Acta Chir. Plast. *11*, 197–209 (1969).

128. Petty, P. G.: Cranioplasty, a Follow-Up Study. Med. J. Austr. *2*, 806–808 (1974).

129. Pfeiffer, R.: Fusion der Wirbelsäule mit dem Autopolymerisat Palacos. Arch. orthop. Unfall-Chir. *62/3*, 250–255 (1967).

130. Pfenninger, J., Kaiser, G.: Die kontinuierliche intrakranielle Drucküberwachung und neue Aspekte in der Neurointensivpflege beim Kind. Schweiz. med. Wschr. *109/44*, 1693–1699 (1979).

131. Pickerill, H. P.: Note on Cranial Autoplasty. Brit. J. Surg. *35*, 204–207 (1948).

132. Pochon, J. P.: The Repair of Congenital and Acquired Skull Defects in Childhood. J. Pediat. Surg. *17/1*, 31–36 (1982).

133. Podvinec, M., Stula, D.: Zur Anwendung alloplastischen Materials bei der Überbrückung frontobasaler Knochendefekte. Aktuelle Probleme der ORL *4*, 91–97. Bern: H. Huber Verlag. 1981.

134. Probst, Ch.: Die plastische Deckung von Schädelkalotten und von frontobasalen Defekten mit frischem autologen Rippenknorpel. Neurochirurgia 16, 105–112 (1973).

135. Pudenz, R. H.: The Repair of Cranial Defects with Tantalum. J.A.M.A. 121/7, 478–481 (1943).

136. Rasmussen, P., Husby, J.: Proceedings of the 28th Annual Meeting of the Nordisk Neurokirurgisk Forening. Acta Neurochir. (Wien) 37, 304–305 (1977).

137. Reeves, D. L.: Cranioplasty. American Lecture Series, Bd. 39. Springfield, Ill.: Ch. C Thomas Publisher. 1950.

138. Richany, S. F., Bast, Th. H., Sprinz, H.: The Repair of Bone and Fate of Autogenous Bone Grafts in the Skull. Acta Neurochir. (Wien) 11, 61–82 (1963).

139. Richard, K. E.: Intrakranielle Drucksteigerung, ihre Pathogenese, Klinik und Behandlung. Nervenarzt 51, 392–405 (1980).

140. Riechert, T.: Über ein neues Verfahren zur Operation des Turmschädels. Zbl. Neurochir. 18/2 and 3, 74–80 (1958).

141. Rietz, K. A.: The One-Stage Method of Cranioplasty with Acrylic Plastic. J. Neurosurg. 15, 176–182 (1958).

142. Rish, B. L., Dillon, J. D., Meirowsky, A. M., Caveness, W. F., Mohr, J. P., Kistler, J. P., Weiss, G. H.: Cranioplasty: A Review of 1030 Cases of Penetrating Head Injury. Neurosurgery 4/5, 381–385 (1979).

143. Röpke, N.: Zur Frage der Deckung von Schädeldefekten. Zbl. Chir. 39, 1192–1194 (1912).

144. Rolle, J.: Über die Verwendung von Klebstoffen in der Medizin. Die Schwester 5, 1968.

145. Rosenmeyer, F. W.: Schnell herstellbare Kunststoffplastik zur Deckung von Schädelknochenlücken. Acta Neurochir. (Wien), Suppl. III, 18–25 (1955).

146. Roth, H.: Die Konservierung von Knochengewebe, pp. 34–68. Wien: Springer. 1952.

147. Schönbauer, L., Winkler, E.: Rekonstruktion von Knochendefekten des Schädels mit Beckenknochen. Zbl. Chir. 16, 672–675 (1954).

148. Schirmer, M.: Einführung in die Neurochirurgie, 4. Aufl., pp. 228–229. Wien-München: Urban & Schwarzenberg. 1979.

149. Schulze, H. E.: Plastischer Verschluß von Schädeldachlücken durch Totknochen. Zbl. Neurochir. 3, 169–176 (1954).

150. Schweiberer, L.: Experimentelle Untersuchungen von Knochentransplantaten mit unveränderter und mit denaturisierter Knochengrundsubstanz. Ein Beitrag zur kausalen Osteogenese. In: Hefte zur Unfallheilkunde (Bürkle de la Camp, C. H., ed.), 103, 3–21. Berlin-Heidelberg-New York: Springer. 1970.

151. Scollo-Lavizzari, G., Matthis, H.: Pharmakologische Grundsätze in der Langzeittherapie der Epilepsien. Schweiz. Rundschau Med. (PRAXIS) 69/14, 443–450 (1980).

152. Scott, M., Wycis, H., Murthagh, F.: Long Term Evaluation of Stainless Steel Cranioplasty. Surg. Gynec. Obstet. 10, 453–461. 1962.

153. Segmüller, G.: Spongiosaregeneration in der Milliporekammer. Helv. chir. Acta 1/2, 5–9 (1967).

154. Seydel: Eine neue Methode, große Knochendefekte des Schädels zu decken. Centralblatt Chir. 12, 209–211 (1889).

155. Staindl, O., Kollar, W. A. F.: Zur Kranioplastik posttraumatischer frontaler Schädellücken. Wien. med. Wschr. 13, 391–393 (1978).

156. Steinhäuser, E. W., Hardt, N.: Neue Aspekte bei der osteoplastischen Rekonstruktion der Schädelkalotte. Méd. et Hyg. 38, 794–799 (1980).

157. Stricker, H.: Der monomere Cyanoacrylsäurebutylester, seine polymerisations-kinetische Charakterisierung und die Entwicklung eines Präparates zur chirurgischen Wundverklebung. Arch. Pharmazie *300*/4, 289–298 (1967).

158. Stula, D.: Schädeldachplastik bei Kindern. Z. Kinderchir. *27*, 297–302 (1979).

159. Stula, D., Müller, H. R.: Schädeldachplastik nach großen dekompressiven Kraniotomien mit Massenverschiebung. CT-Analyse. Neurochirurgia *23*, 41–46 (1980).

160. Stula, D.: Rekonstruktive Eingriffe bei ausgedehnten posttraumatischen Schädel-defekten. Aktuelle Probleme der Otorhinologie, pp. 106–111. Bern: H. Huber. 1981.

161. Stula, D.: The Problem of the "Sinking Skin Flap Syndrome" in Cranioplasty. J. max.-fac. Surg. *10*/3, 142–145 (1982).

162. Tabaddor, K., LaMorgese, J.: Complication of a Large Cranial Defect. J. Neurosurg. *44*, 506–508 (1976).

163. Thomalske, G.: Die plastische Deckung von Schädelknochendefekten im Schnell-verfahren nach Woringer. Med. Bild-Dienst 2, Juni 1962.

164. Thomson, H. G., Hoffman, H. J.: Intracranial Use of a Breast Prosthesis to Temporarily Stabilize a Reduction Cranioplasty. Plast. Reconstr. Surg. *55*/6, 704–707 (1975).

165. Timmons, R. L.: Cranial Defects and Their Repair. Neurolog. Surgery II, 993–1008. Philadelphia-London-Toronto: W. B. Saunders. 1973.

166. Uehlinger, E., Puls, P.: Funktionelle Anpassung des Knochens auf physiologische und unphysiologische Beanspruchung. Langenbecks Arch. klin. Chir. *319*, 362–374 (1967).

167. Uemura, K., Yamaura, A., Makino, H.: The Syndrome of Intracranial Hypertension. Traumatology (Tokyo) *6*, 387–392 (1975).

168. Umbach, W.: Zur Behandlung des chronischen intraduralen Hämatoms. Langenbecks Arch. klin. Chir. *287*, 666–669 (1957).

169. Unger, R. R., Sollmann, H.: Die Versorgung von Schädelkalottendefekten mit Palacos. Zbl. Chir. *23*, 850–856 (1964).

170. Van Meekren, J.: Observations medicochirurgical. 392, 6 pl. Amsterdam: Henrici and T. Bloom. 1682.

171. Venable, C. S., Stuck, W. G.: A General Consideration of Metal for Buried Applicances in Surgery. Surg. Gynec. Obstet. *76*, 297–304 (1943).

172. Vinken, P. J., Bruyn, G. W.: Handbook of Clinical Neurology, pp. 105–113. Amsterdam: North-Holland Publishing *17*/3. 1975.

173. Vogt, G.: Plastischer Verschluß knöcherner Schädellücken mit Kunststoff-prothesen. Acta Neurochir. (Wien), Suppl. III, 26–30 (1955).

174. Wagner, A., Umbach, W.: Die plastische Deckung von knöchernen Schädel-defekten. Dtsch. Med. J. *7*, 191–197 (1963).

175. Wahlig, H., Hameister, W., Grieben, A.: Über die Freisetzung von Gentamycin aus Polymethylmethacrylat. Langenbecks Arch. Chir. *331*, 169–192 (1972).

176. Wahlig, H., Buchholz, H. W.: Experimentelle und klinische Untersuchungen zur Freisetzung von Gentamycin aus einem Knochenzement. Chirurg *43*, 441–445 (1972).

177. Walkter, A. E., Jablon, S.: A Follow-Up Study of Head Wounds in World War II, p. 202. Washington, D. C.: U.S. Government Printing Office. 1961.

178. Weiford, E. C., Gardner, W. J.: Tantalum Cranioplasty. Review of 106 Cases in Civilian Practice. J. Neurosurg. *6*, 13–32 (1949).

179. Werner, A.: Deux cas d'emparrure ouverte du sinus frontal avec hacération meningée. Plastique cranienne avec résine. Praxis *32*, 735 (1955).

180. White, R. J., Yashon, D., Albin, M. S., Wilson, D.: Delayed Acrylic Reconstruction of the Skull in Craniocerebral Trauma. J. Traumat. *10*/9, 780–786 (1970).

181. Wiedemann, K., Hamer, J., Weinhardt, F., Just, O. H.: Barbituratinfusion bei schwerem Schädelhirntrauma. Anästh. intensivther. Notfallmed. *15*, 303–314 (1980).

182. Wölfel, J. D.: Vom Sinn der Trepanation. Ciba Zeitschr. *39*, 1326–1331 (1936).

183. Woringer, E., Schwieg, B., Brogly, G., Schneider, J.: Nouvelle technique ultra-rapide pour la réfection de brèches osseuses craniennes à la résine acrylique. Rev. Neurol. *85*/6, 527–535 (1951).

184. Woringer, E., Thomalske, G.: Über die plastische Deckung von Schädelknochen-defekten mit autopolymerisierender Kunstharzmasse. – Eine neue Schnell-methode. Arch. Psychiat. u. Z. Neurol. *191*, 100–113 (1953).

185. Yamada, H., Sakai, N., Takada, M., Ando, T., Kagawa, Y.: Cranioplasty Utilizing a Preserved Autogenous Bone Flap Coated with Acrylic Resin. Acta Neurochir. (Wien) *52*, 273–280 (1980).

186. Yamaura, A., Makino, H.: Neurological Deficits in the Presence of the Sinking Skin Flap Following Decompressive Craniectomy. Neurol. medico Chir. *17*, 43–53 (1977).

187. Yamaura, A., Sato, M., Meguro, K., Nakamura, T., Uemura, K., Makino, H.: Cranioplasty Following Decompressive Craniectomy. Analysis of 300 Cases. Neurolog. Surg. (Tokyo) *5*/4, 345–353 (1977).

188. Zeidler, U., Kottke, S., Hundeshagen, H., (eds.): Hirnszintigraphie, Technik und Klinik, pp. 207–208: Hirnszintigraphie bei Knochenprozessen; pp. 214–217: Prae- und postoperative Diagnostik. Berlin-Heidelberg-New York: Springer. 1972.

Index

To be published in Winter 1984

Microsurgery of Cerebral Veins

By Professor **Wolfgang Seeger,** Medical Director of the Department of General Neurosurgery and Chairman of Neurosurgery of the Neurosurgical Clinic, University of Freiburg i. Br.

1984. Approx. 200 figures. Approx. 420 pages.
ISBN 3-211-81807-3

Contrary to brain arteries, cerebral veins are positioned predominantly on the brain surface which includes the deeply penetrating dura duplicatures (Falx and Tentorium). The operative approach to deeper brainstructures is often hindered by large veins. Even today it remains impossible to verify before the operation precisely whether the interruption of specific large or small veins may be carried out without risking neurological and/or psychic deficiencies, although veins anastomose more extensively than arteries. It has long been known that sudden operative interruption of Sinus longitudinalis sup. in its middle or posterior portions may be fatal. Less known are the often harmless consequences of interrupting larger cerebral veins of the brain convexity. In the present volume cerebral veins are described solely from the viewpoint of operative technique. It shows you the technical possibilities for sparing the venous collateral circulation where the original veins and Sinus are interrupted by tumor. As Dr. Seeger's previous books, "Microsurgery of the Cerebral Veins" stresses topographical anatomical viewpoints and microsurgical techniques. Ophthalmologists will find special value in the descriptions of the venous connections to the Ala major, ossis sphenoidalis and Fissura orbitalis sup. Otorhinolaryngologists will be interested in the particular situations involving Sinus sigmoideus, while neuropathologists and neuroradiologists will find the problematic operative procedures in the area of cerebral veins—as shown from the surgeon's viewpoint—to be particularly relevant.

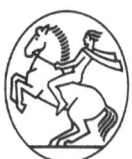

Springer-Verlag Wien NewYork